Pocket Picture Guides
for Nurses

Pediatrics

Pocket Picture Guides
for Nurses

Pediatrics

Ian W. Booth   BSc, MSc, MB BS, MRCP (UK),
DObst RCOG, DCH

Lecturer, Institute of Child Health,
London, UK
Honorary Senior Registrar,
The Hospital for Sick Children,
Great Ormond Street, London, UK

Edward R. Wozniak   BSc, MB BS, MRCP, DCH

Research Fellow, Institute of Child Health,
London, UK
Honorary Senior Registrar,
The Hospital for Sick Children,
Great Ormond Street, London, UK

Williams & Wilkins Baltimore London

Western Hemisphere distribution rights held by
Williams and Wilkins
428 East Preston Street
Baltimore, MD 21202, USA

ISBN 0-683-00922-2

Library of Congress Cataloging in Publication Data
Booth, I.
    Pediatrics.
    (Pocket picture guides for nurses)
    1. Children—Diseases—Diagnosis—Atlases.
I. Wozniak, E. II. Title. III. Series. [DNLM:
1. Occupational therapy. 2. Models, Theoretical.
WY 17 B725p]
RJ50.B66 1984   618.92'0075   83-7041

Project Editor: Fiona Carr
    Designer: Teresa Foster

Originated in Hong Kong by Imago Publishing Ltd.
Printed in Great Britain by W. S. Cowell Ltd.

Pocket Picture Guides
for Nurses

The purpose of this series is to provide essential visual
information about commonly encountered diseases in a
convenient practical and economic format. Each Pocket
Picture Guide covers an important area of day-to-day
clinical medicine. The main feature of these books is the
superbly photographed colour reproductions of typical
clinical appearances. Other visual diagnostic
information, such as X-rays, is included where
appropriate. Each illustration is fully explained by a
clearly written descriptive caption highlighting important
diagnostic features. Tables presenting other diagnostic
and differential diagnostic information are included
where appropriate. A comprehensive and carefully
compiled index makes each Pocket Picture Guide an easy
to use source of visual reference.

An extensive series is planned and other titles in the
initial group of Pocket Picture Guides are:

Infectious Diseases
Rheumatic Diseases
Sexually Transmitted Diseases
Skin Diseases

To Chloe and Alexander; Hannah and Michael

Contents

Introduction

This collection of colour clinical photographs is intended as a supplement to standard paediatric texts. Within the limitations of its size, we have tried to include as many common childhood conditions as possible. Several uncommon conditions have been included; those which demonstrate particular physical signs and those in which early recognition will influence management. We hope that this book will therefore be useful to undergraduate and postgraduate students of paediatrics and paediatric nursing.

We are grateful to the staff of the Hospital for Sick Children, Great Ormond Street, London and in particular Mr. R. Lunnon and Mr. M. Johns in the Department of Medical Illustration for providing an extensive library of high quality clinical photographs from which all these photographs were taken, except where indicated. Our thanks go to those who have kindly provided additional photographs.

The Neonate

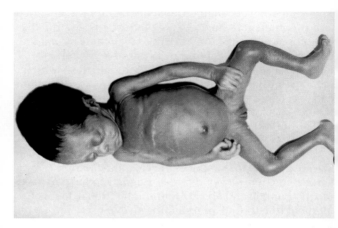

Fig. 1   Pre-term infant. The upper limbs are extended with frog-like flexion of the lower limbs. The labia majora are separated with the labia minora protruding. The skin is thin and translucent. By courtesy of TALC, Institute of Child Health.

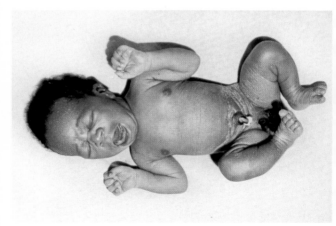

Fig. 2   Full term infant. In contrast to the pre-term infant there is full flexion of the knees, hips and elbows and the genitalia are mature. The skin is thicker and more subcutaneous fat is present. By courtesy of TALC, Institute of Child Health.

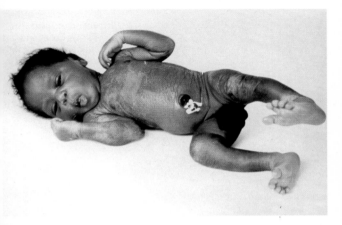

Fig. 3 Post-mature infant. The gestation period is over 42 weeks and the infant has characteristically dry, peeling skin. By courtesy of TALC, Institute of Child Health.

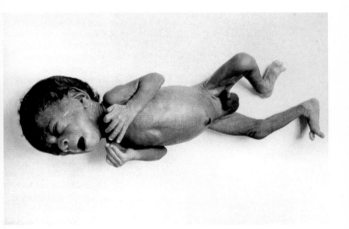

Fig. 4 Light-for-dates infant. This term baby weighed only 1.7 kg. The head appears disproportionately large for the thin, wasted body. This results from placental insufficiency late in pregnancy. Hypoglycaemia may be a complication. By courtesy of TALC, Institute of Child Health.

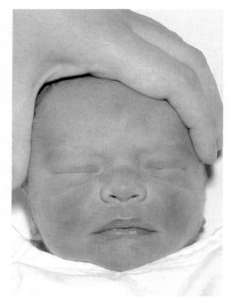

Fig. 5 Face to pubes presentation. There is extensive bruising and petechiae of the presenting part. The infant is not cyanosed. Extensive neonatal bruising may result in jaundice.

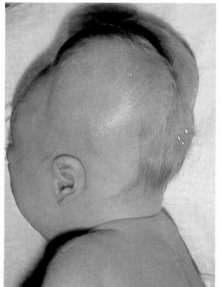

Fig. 6 Cephalhaematoma. Swellings are present over both parietal bones. These are subperiosteal haemorrhages which may be associated with skull fracture. Jaundice may develop. Spontaneous resolution occurs, sometimes with calcification. By courtesy of Dr. P. Daish and by kind permission of Dr. P.M. Dunn.

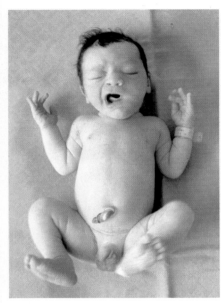

Fig. 7 Facial palsy. A left facial palsy is present in this term baby. This is a lower motor neurone lesion which may result from pressure *in utero* or following forceps delivery. If the nerve fibres are not torn, recovery occurs after a few weeks but the eye may need special care during this time. By courtesy of Dr. P. Daish and by kind permission of Dr. P.M. Dunn.

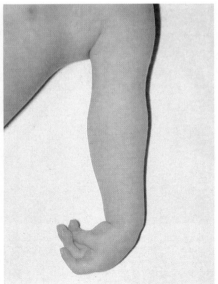

Fig. 8 Erb's palsy. The arm is internally rotated, with pronation of the forearm and the characteristic 'waiter's tip' position of the hand. This C5-6 branchial plexus lesion is often due to shoulder traction during delivery.

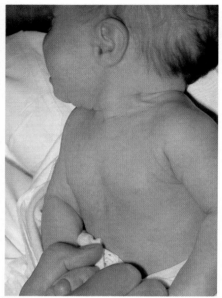

Fig. 9
Sternomastoid tumour. There is shortening of the left sternocleidomastoid with swelling in its mid portion. The condition is of unknown aetiology and is associated with torticollis if untreated.

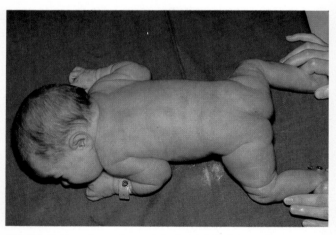

Fig. 10 Toxic erythema (neonatal urticaria). Blotchy erythema occurs with firm yellow-white pustules. These contain eosinophil-rich fluid which is sterile on culture. This condition is common, benign and self-limiting and usually appears around the second day of life.

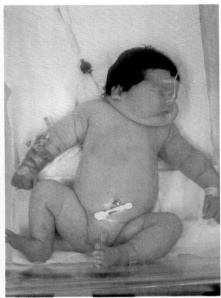

Fig. 11 Infant of diabetic mother. These babies are large and fat, often over 4 kg, and all look remarkably similar. Visceromegaly may be present. Early hypoglycaemia is common and there is an increased incidence of hyaline membrane disease, cardiac failure and hypocalcaemia. By By courtesy of Dr. P. Daish and by kind permission of Dr. P.M. Dunn.

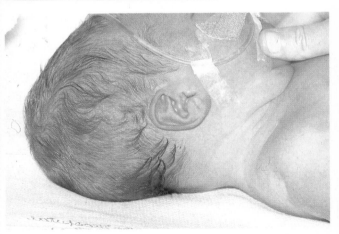

Fig. 12 Beckwith's syndrome. These infants are of high birth weight with macroglossia, exomphalos (see Fig. 178) and visceromegaly. Characteristic linear creases are present in the ear lobe. Hypoglycaemia is common and may be severe and persistent.

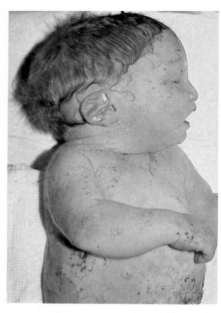

Fig. 13 Potter's syndrome. Bilateral renal agenesis results in oligohydramnios with fetal compression. Pulmonary hypoplasia is present. There are characteristically low-set ears, a receding chin and beaked nose. Such infants are frequently stillborn, or die in the early neonatal period.

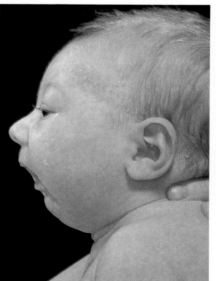

Fig. 14 Pierre-Robin syndrome. Mandibular hypoplasia leads to posterior displacement of the tongue, and a rounded palatal cleft. Obstruction of the upper airways may occur but this can be relieved by bringing the tongue forward. Feeding requires extra patience. Growth results in a normal profile.

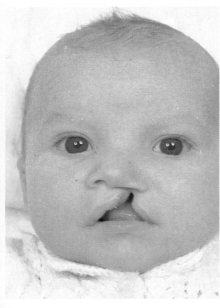

Fig. 15 Unilateral cleft lip. The alveolar margin is usually involved, and the nose is displaced and deformed. This condition may be associated with a cleft palate. The lip is usually repaired at around two months of age.

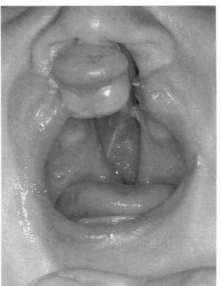

Fig. 16 Bilateral cleft lip and palate. The cleft extends from the soft to the hard palate, exposing the nasal cavity. Protrusion of the intermaxillary process is present. A multidisciplinary approach to management is important, as speech and dental problems arise in addition to the obvious cosmetic ones.

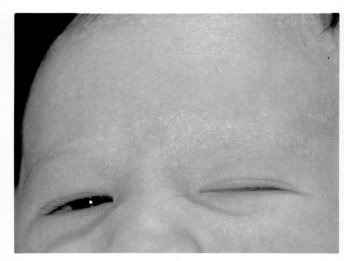

Fig. 17 Seborrhoeic dermatitis. A dry, scaly, non-pruritic erythematous dermatitis is seen, which may begin in the first month of life and is common throughout the first year. It affects the scalp (see Fig. 153), face, neck and napkin area.

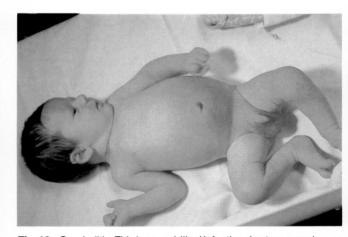

Fig. 18 Omphalitis. This is an umbilical infection due to pyogenic bacteria and is a serious complication of the neonatal period. Spread of infection to the liver or haematogenous spread are potentially serious complications which can be prevented by correct umbilical care. By courtesy of Dr. P. Daish.

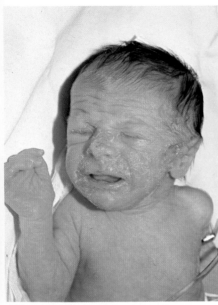

Fig. 19 Ritter's disease (toxic epidermal necrolysis; scalded skin syndrome). This is an infection by an exo-toxin producing *Staphylococcus aureus* which affects infants and young children. The skin is erythematous and tender; flaccid bullae appear and there is crusting around the mouth.

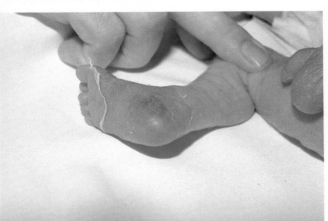

Fig. 20 Ritter's disease. Large sheets of epidermis readily peel away, leaving areas which quickly dry and heal within two to three days. Prompt, systemic, penicillinase-resistant antibiotic treatment is essential.

10

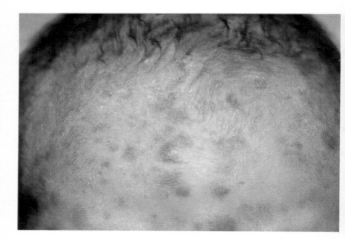

Fig. 21 Neonatal purpura. Small superficial haemorrhages are present in the skin, due to thrombocytopenia. This may be caused by infections (especially congenital rubella or cytomegalovirus) or by placental transfer of anti-platelet antibodies in maternal idiopathic thrombocytopenic purpura.

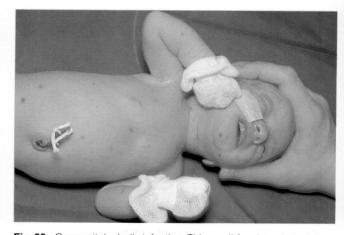

Fig. 22 Congenital rubella infection. This small-for-dates baby has neonatal hepatitis with hepatomegaly, conjugated-hyperbilirubinaemia and purpura. The central nervous system is involved, resulting in opisthotonus. Other features may include interstitial pneumonia, congenital heart disease, skeletal abnormalities, retinopathy and cataract (see Fig. 70).

11

Congenital Malformations

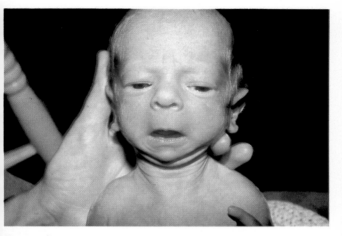

Fig. 23 Fetal-alcohol syndrome. Alcohol is the most common teratogenic agent to which the fetus is exposed. Prenatal growth deficiency, short palpebral fissures, a smooth philtrum and a thin smooth upper lip are characteristic. By courtesy of the Dept. of Genetics, Institute of Child Health.

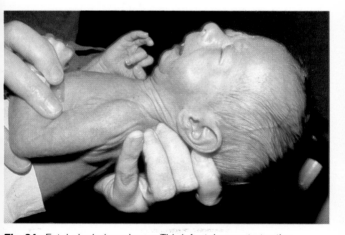

Fig. 24 Fetal-alcohol syndrome. This infant demonstrates the maxillary hypoplasia present in this syndrome. The ears appear relatively large due to microcephaly. By courtesy of the Dept. of Genetics, Institute of Child Health.

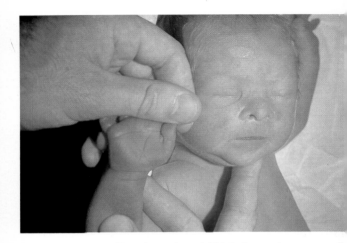

Fig. 25 Trisomy 21 (Down's syndrome). This is the most common chromosomal abnormality (1 in 660 newborn). This infant has a flat facial profile, slanted palpebral fissures and a Simian crease (present in only half of these infants). Hypotonia, a poorly developed Moro reflex and hyperextendable joints are usual. The auricles are often anomalous and there is redundant skin on the back of the neck. By courtesy of Dr. B. D. Speidel

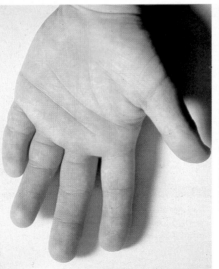

Fig. 26 Trisomy 21 (Down's syndrome). The metacarpals and phalanges are relatively short, resulting in square, stubby hands. Hypoplasia of the mid-phalanx of the fifth finger with incurving is present. The single palmar crease (Simian crease) is not present. By courtesy of the Dept. of Genetics, Institute of Child Health.

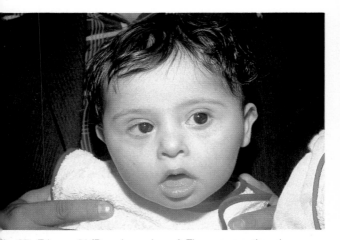

Fig. 27 Trisomy 21 (Down's syndrome). The open mouth and protruding tongue result from hypotonia. There is a low nasal bridge with a tendency to epicanthic folds. By courtesy of the Dept. of Genetics, Institute of Child Health.

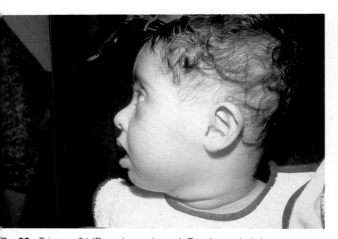

Fig. 28 Trisomy 21 (Down's syndrome). Brachycephaly is present (shortened anteroposterior skull diameter and flattened occiput) and the hair is sparse. By courtesy of the Dept. of Genetics, Insitute of Child Health.

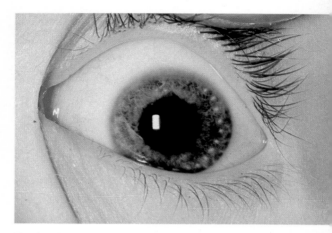

Fig. 29 Trisomy 21 (Down's syndrome). Speckling of the iris is present (Brushfield spots). Refractive errors may occur and lens opacities may be seen on slit-lamp examination. By courtesy of TALC Institute of Child Health.

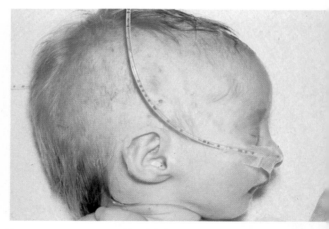

Fig. 30 Trisomy 18 (Edward's syndrome). This is the second most common chromosomal abnormality (1 in 3,000 newborn). There is a prominent occiput with low-set, malformed auricles and a small mouth and chin. 90% of cases die in the first year of life and the remainder are mentally retarded.

15

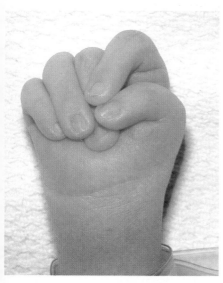

Fig. 31 Trisomy 18 (Edward's syndrome). The hand is clenched with the index finger overlapping the third finger. The nails are hypoplastic.

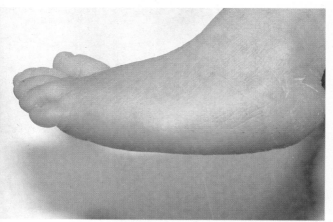

Fig. 32 Trisomy 18 (Edward's syndrome). The hallux is short and dorsiflexed. The foot has a characteristic 'rocker bottom' appearance.

16

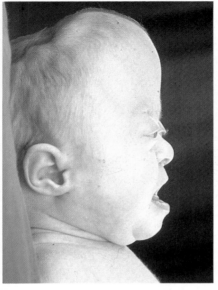

Fig. 33 Craniofacial dysostosis (Crouzon's syndrome). There is premature fusion of the skull sutures (craniosynostosis) with visible ridging. The anteroposterior diameter of the skull is short, with shallow orbits, ocular proptosis, a hypoplastic maxilla and a beaked nose. Optic atrophy may develop. Inheritance is autosomal dominant with variable expression.

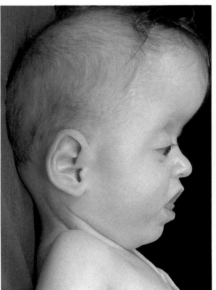

Fig. 34 Acrocephalo-syndactyly (Apert's syndrome). Craniosynostosis of the coronal suture results in a high pointed head (acrocephaly) with a full forehead, flat occiput and flat facies. Syndactyly of fingers and toes occurs and non-skeletal congenital abnormalities are common.

17

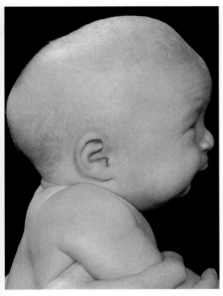

Fig. 35
Scaphocephaly. The head is elongated due to premature fusion of the sagittal suture preventing lateral growth of the skull. Abnormal expansion superiorly and in the anteroposterior axis results. Ocular and neurological abnormalities are rare.

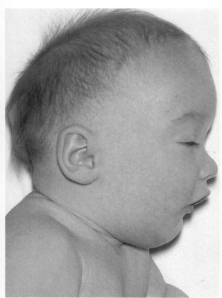

Fig. 36
Brachycephaly. The occiput is flat and there is anteroposterior shortening and increased height of the skull. These appearances result from craniosynostosis of the lambdoid sutures, which may be palpable.

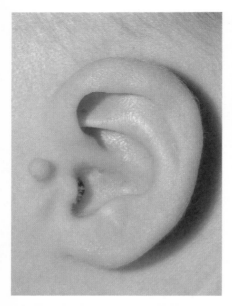

Fig. 37 Pre-auricular tag. This may occur as an isolated lesion or in association with anomalies of the face and ears. Skin tags on a narrow pedicle can be ligated, otherwise surgical excision is required.

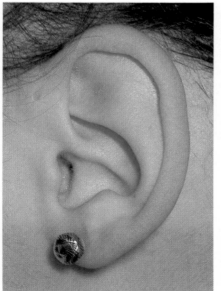

Fig. 38 Pre-auricular sinus. This results from imperfect fusion of the first two branchial arches. It may be associated with other anomalies of the face and ears. Chronic infection can occur, requiring excision.

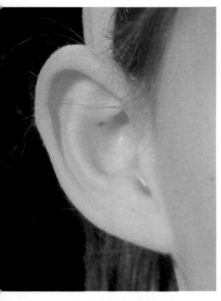

Fig. 39 Jug ear. Failure of formation of the antihelix results in a prominent ear. Surgical correction is best undertaken at four or five years; earlier operation may result in recurrence.

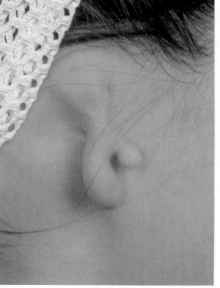

Fig. 40 Microtia. This rudimentary auricle results from early developmental abnormalities in the first and second branchial arches. It is associated with severe abnormalities of the middle ear and may also be associated with other craniofacial and renal abnormalities.

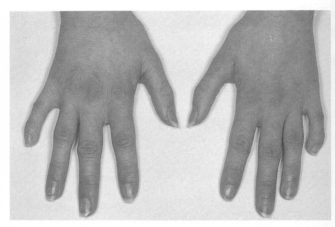

Fig. 41 Clinodactyly. There is incurving of the fifth finger which is abnormally short. This may be seen in many congenital syndromes including trisomy 21 and Russell-Silver dwarfism.

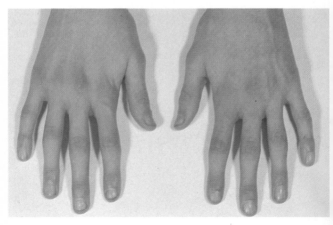

Fig. 42 Arachnodactyly. Abnormally long, tapering fingers are a feature of Marfan's syndrome, homocystinuria and other conditions.

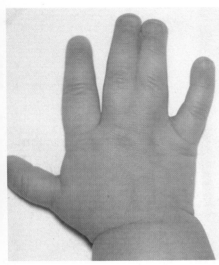

Fig. 43 Syndactyly. The soft tissues of the third and fourth digits are fused. Bony fusion may also occur. This condition may be present in a variety of combinations and degrees of severity in several congenital syndromes. Surgical separation is required for normal growth of the digits.

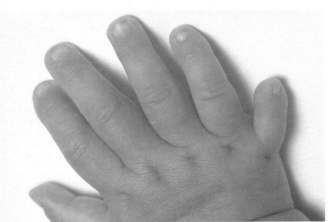

Fig. 44 Polydactyly. This may be familial and associated with a number of congenital syndromes. If the extra digit contains bone its removal should be delayed until ossification can be defined, towards the end of the first year.

22

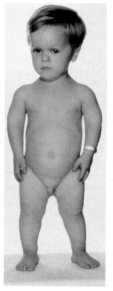
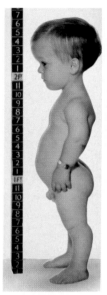

Fig. 45
Achondroplasia. There is short stature with a large head, low nasal bridge, prominent forehead, lumbar lordosis and short limbs. Spinal complications are common and long-term follow-up is required. Inheritance is autosomal dominant, but most cases are fresh mutations (sometimes with elderly fathers).

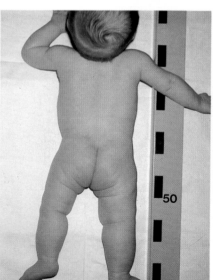

Fig. 46
Hemihypertrophy. This child has hemihypertrophy with obvious enlargement of the right lower limb. It may be associated with mental retardation, Wilms' tumour, adrenal carcinoma or Silver's syndrome. Organs on the same side may be similarly affected.

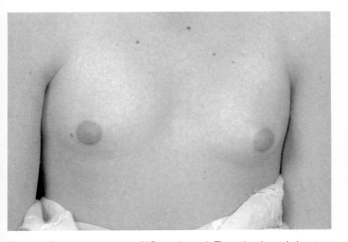

Fig. 47 Turner's syndrome (XO syndrome). There is a broad chest with widely-spaced nipples. Breast development can occur in XO/XX mosaics but is usually as a result of oestrogen replacement therapy in late adolescence. Short stature and gonadal dysgenesis are usual. Renal, skeletal and cardiac abnormalities are common.

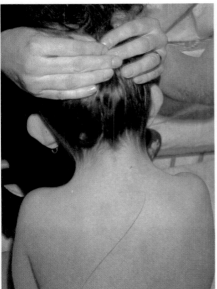

Fig. 48 Turner's syndrome (XO syndrome). Webbing of the neck and a low, 'trident' hairline are present. The presence of lymphoedema of the digits during the neonatal period may help in the diagnosis of this syndrome.

Ear, Nose and Throat and the Respiratory System

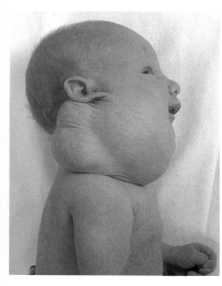

Fig. 49 Cystic hygroma. There is a large lymphangiomatous swelling of the face and neck. The mass is fluctuant and transilluminates. It may cause obstruction of the upper airways at birth or in later life, due to enlargement during upper respiratory tract infections or haemorrhage into the lesion.

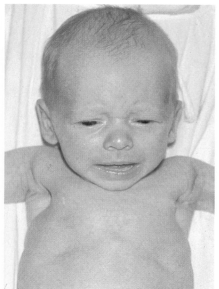

Fig. 50 Congenital laryngeal stridor. Weakness of the upper airways causes stridor from birth. This may change with posture and improves with age. When severe, intercostal recession and feeding difficulties occur. Direct laryngoscopy may be required to exclude other malformations.

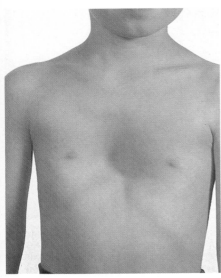

Fig. 51 Funnel chest (pectus excavatum). This is usually congenital but may follow chronic respiratory obstruction or rickets. Cardiopulmonary embarrassment is unusual.

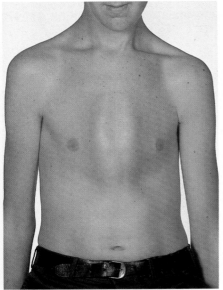

Fig. 52 Pigeon chest. The sternum and costal cartilages are prominent. Muscle or breast development at puberty tends to obscure the abnormality.

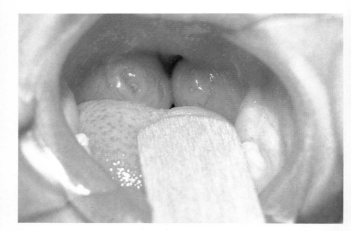

Fig. 53 Tonsillitis. The tonsils are enlarged, hyperaemic, superficially ulcerated and meet in the midline. In association with adenoidal hypertrophy, this may result in significant upper airways obstruction. Gagging during examination may draw the tonsils forward leading to artefactual hypertrophy.

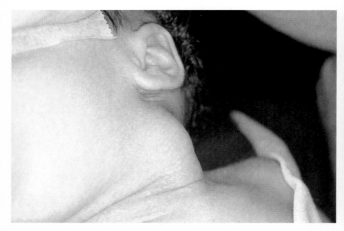

Fig. 54 Lymphadenopathy. A solitary enlarged cervical lymph node may occur as a result of local sepsis, tuberculosis, atypical mycobacterial infection or malignancy.

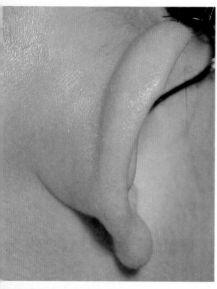

Fig. 55 Mastoiditis. Infection of the mastoid air cells, usually from otitis media, has produced overlying erythema and oedema, resulting in the forward and downward displacement of the external ear. Osteitis should be managed surgically.

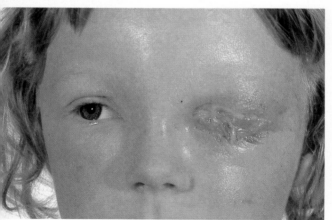

Fig. 56 Orbital cellulitis. Infection in and around the tissues of the orbit may result from spread of infection from paranasal sinuses or the face. The eyelids are inflamed and swollen and eye movement may be impaired. Cavernous sinus thrombosis, blindness or meningitis may result.

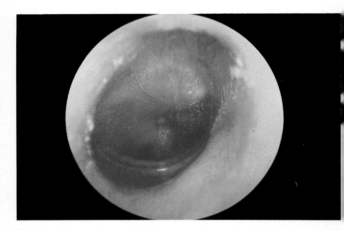

Fig. 57 Acute otitis media. The tympanic membrane is inflamed and bulging forwards, with loss of the light reflex. This followed an upper respiratory tract infection and the child presented with screaming and fever. Perforation may occur, resulting in discharge from the ear and relief of pain. By courtesy of the Dept. of Medical Illustration, University of Aberdeen.

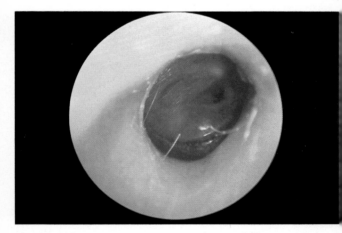

Fig. 58 Chronic secondary otitis media (glue ear). The tympanic membrane is dull, slate-coloured and bulging forwards with a fluid level visible. These changes are associated with a conductive hearing loss which is usually bilateral. Blockage of the Eustachian tube due to adenoidal hypertrophy may be an aetiological factor. By courtesy of the Dept. of Medical Illustration, University of Aberdeen.

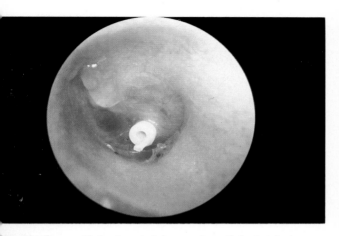

Fig. 59 Grommet in treatment of glue ear. A small plastic tube has been inserted through the tympanic membrane, following drainage of fluid in the middle ear. This preserved aeration and prevented reaccumulation of fluid in a child with persistent glue ears and deafness. Rapid improvement in hearing occurred. By courtesy of the Dept. of Medical Illustration, University of Aberdeen.

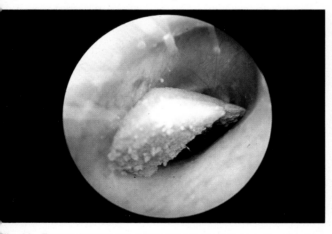

Fig. 60 Foreign body in ear. A fragment of an eraser was found to be present in the external auditory canal of this child with otitis media. Removal of foreign bodies should not be carried out by the unskilled as damage to the tympanic membrane may occur. By courtesy of the Dept. of Medical Illustration, University of Aberdeen.

The Eye

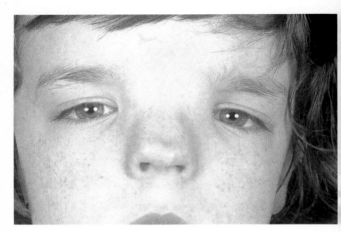

Fig. 61 Hypertelorism. There is increased interpupillary distance (standard measurements available) with apparent broadening of the bridge of the nose. This may be associated with mental retardation and a number of syndromes including chromosomal anomalies.

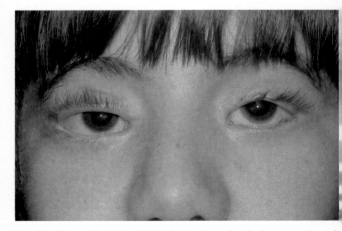

Fig. 62 Epicanthic folds. A fold of skin obscuring the inner canthus of the eye is present, which may give the impression of a squint. The fold disappears with growth of the bridge of the nose. Epicanthic folds are commonly seen in normal infants and are also seen in trisomy 21 and other syndromes.

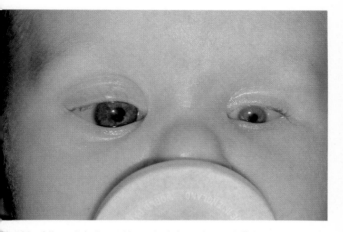

Fig. 63 Microphthalmos. Here, the left eye is small. This can be unilateral or bilateral and may be genetically determined. Other ocular abnormalities may occur in addition, including coloboma and cataract.

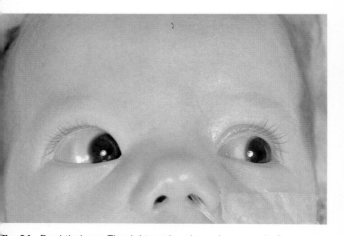

Fig. 64 Buphthalmos. The right eye is enlarged as a result of increased intra-ocular pressure (infantile glaucoma). This is the most common cause of a large eye in infancy and requires urgent ophthalmological management to prevent blindness.

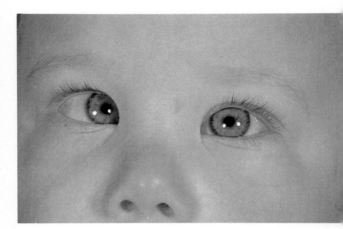

Fig. 65 Squint. A right convergent non-paralytic (concomitant) squint is present. The deviation is constant in all directions of gaze and the reflected light from the cornea is asymmetrical. Early ophthalmological referral is required to prevent loss of vision in the squinting eye.

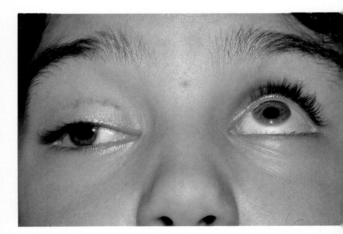

Fig. 66 Third nerve palsy. A paralytic squint is present, with downward and outward deviation of the right eye whatever the direction of gaze of the left. The right pupil is enlarged and a right ptosis is present.

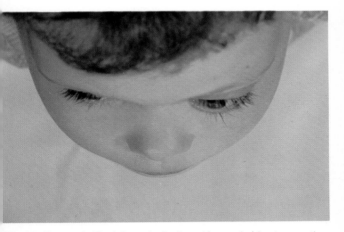

Fig. 67 Proptosis. The left eye is displaced forwards (due to an optic nerve glioma). The asymmetry of the orbits may be best visualised from above. Unilateral lesions are usually due to neoplasms, particularly metastatic neuroblastoma. Vascular lesions may produce an orbital bruit.

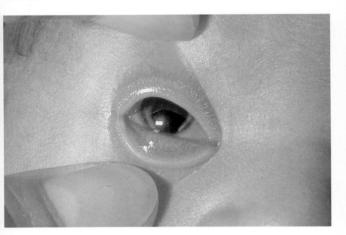

Fig. 68 Coloboma. A sector defect is present in the lower part of the iris. A similar defect was present in the retina of this patient (see Fig. 76). By courtesy of Dr. P. Daish and by kind permission of Dr. P M. Dunn.

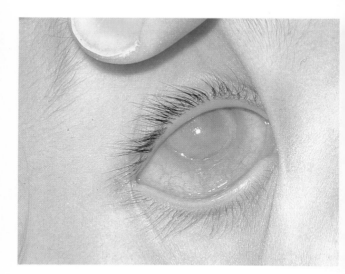

Fig. 69 Corneal opacity. The cornea is cloudy and the red reflex would be absent. Opacification may be seen in some mucopolysaccharidoses or following keratitis or trauma.

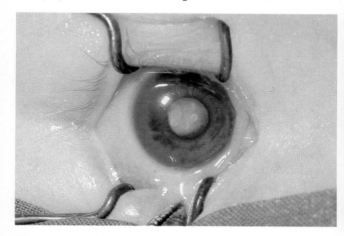

Fig. 70 Cataract. A dense, complete lens opacity is present and a white area now fills the pupil. In this case, the cataract is due to congenital rubella. They may also be secondary to galactosaemia, retrolental fibroplasia, hypercalcaemia, trisomy 21 or steroids.

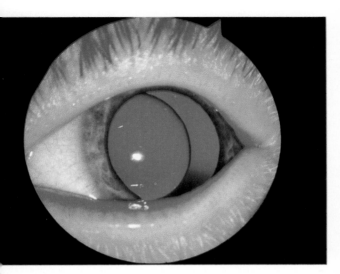

Fig. 71 Lens dislocation. Full pupillary dilatation reveals the presence of a dislocated lens in a patient with Marfan's syndrome. It may also occur in homocystinuria and presents as a refractive error.

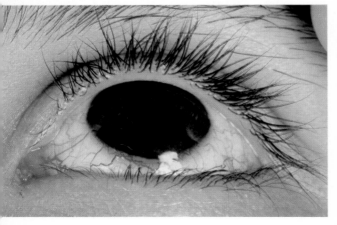

Fig. 72 Ataxia-telangiectasia. Telangiectases are present on the bulbar conjunctiva. This is an autosomal recessive disorder characterised by progressive ataxia, telangiectasia, mental retardation and an immunodeficiency.

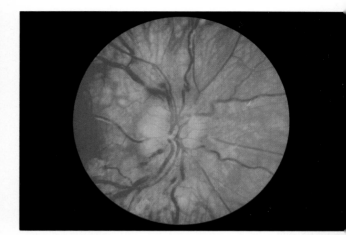

Fig. 73 Papilloedema. The optic disc is congested, its outline blurred and the vessels course upwards over the swollen disc margin. The veins are distended and haemorrhages are present. Papilloedema results from raised intracranial pressure due to tumours, hydrocephalus, encephalopathies or from hypertension.

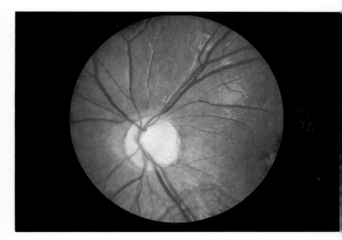

Fig. 74 Optic atrophy. The optic disc is white and clearly demarcated from the fundus due to irreparable damage of the optic nerve which resulted in visual loss. This may be inherited or occur following chronically raised intracranial pressure.

37

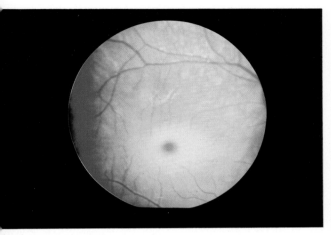

Fig. 75 Tay-Sachs disease. The retina is pale due to lipid storage and degeneration. At the macula the vascular choroid is visible through the retina as a cherry-red spot. This lipid storage disorder is inherited in an autosomal recessive fashion and is characterised by progressive dementia and blindness.

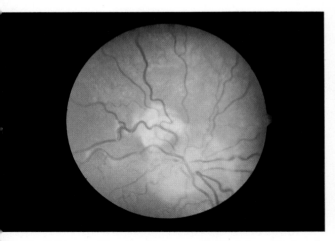

Fig. 76 Coloboma of the choroid. As a result of the failure of fusion of the fetal cleft, an area of choroid bordering the optic disc is missing and white sclera is visible through the defect. The iris (see Fig. 68), optic disc or eyelids may be similarly affected.

The Genitourinary System

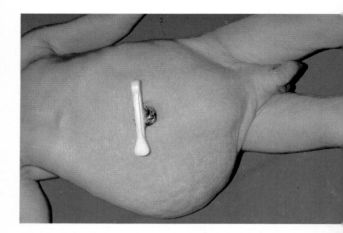

Fig. 77 Prune-belly syndrome. Congenital absence of the muscles of the anterior abdominal wall results in markedly wrinkled skin. This is commonly associated with abnormalities of the urinary tract, such as hypoplastic kidneys, hydronephros, hydroureter, megacystis or intestinal malrotation. It is usually seen in boys.

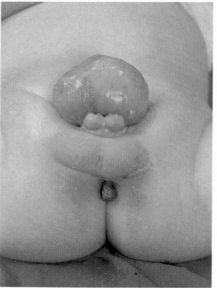

Fig. 78 Bladder extrophy. The bladder is exposed and the penis is characteristically shortened with complete epispadias. The ureteric orifices may be seen in the centre of the mass. The bladder mucosa is very sensitive and tender. Urinary tract infection, vesico-ureteric reflux and hydronephrosis may occur, resulting in renal damage.

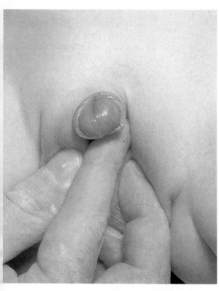

Fig. 79 Epispadias. The dorsal part of the urethra fails to fuse, resulting in a urethral opening above the shaft of the penis. This may be associated with incontinence, which improves with urethral reconstruction at three to four years.

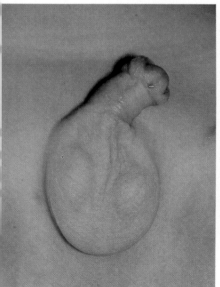

Fig. 80
Hypospadias. The external urethral meatus is on the ventral surface of the glans, but less commonly may open on the shaft of the penis. There may be associated ventral curvature of the shaft of the penis (chordee). Surgical treatment is required for chordee and for urethral openings on the shaft. The hood-shaped prepuce should be preserved until reconstruction is complete.

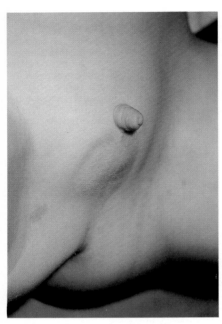

Fig. 81 Micropenis. The penis is very small and cryptorchidism (bilateral undescended testes) is also present. It may be associated with Noonan's or Prader-Willi syndromes.

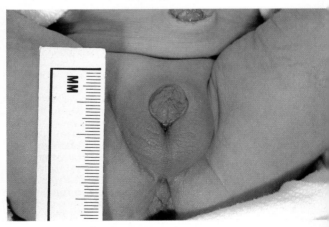

Fig. 82 Ambiguous genitalia. Examination of the external genitalia of this child does not permit sex determination. This patient is female with a large phallus and fused, rugose labia. The commonest cause of female pseudohermaphroditism is congenital adrenal hyperplasia.

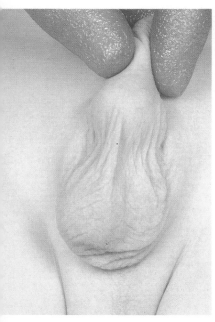

Fig. 83
Undescended left testicle. The left testicle is not present in the scrotum and could not be palpated in the external inguinal canal. The usual management is early orchidopexy.

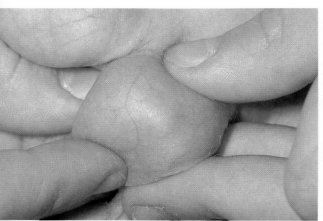

Fig. 84 Torsion of a hydatid cyst of Morgagni. A blue tender swelling is present at the base of the left testis. Pain in the testes of acute onset may also be due to testicular torsion or, less commonly, orchitis.

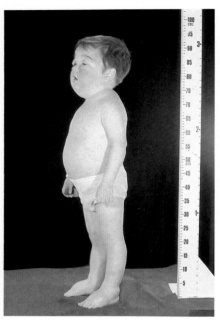

Fig. 85 Nephrotic syndrome. The child has marked generalised oedema and abdominal distention resulting from ascites. Heavy proteinuria results in hypoalbuminaemia, hypovolaemia and secondary hyperaldosteronism. Most cases in childhood are due to a minimal change glomerular lesion and are steroid responsive.

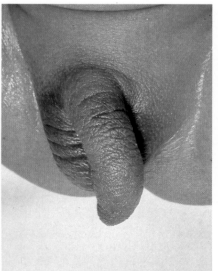

Fig. 86 Congenital adrenal hyperplasia. The penis is enlarged due to 21-hydroxylase deficiency. In the female, the same disorder presents with ambiguous genitalia. Approximately one-third of patients with 21-hydroxylase deficiency are 'salt-losers'. By courtesy of Dr. B. D. Speidel.

The Endocrine System

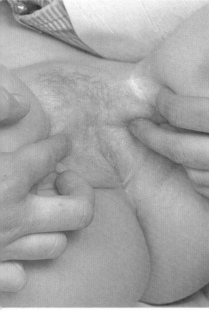

Fig. 87 Premature pubarche. Hair is present on the labia and pubic region of this toddler. This may occur in the absence of the development of other secondary sexual characteristics, which distinguishes this anomaly from true precocious puberty.

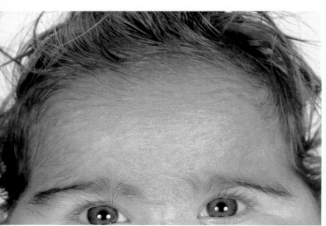

Fig. 88 Cushing's syndrome. The skin of this 21 month old girl is irsute and acne is present. The face is plethoric and obese. The ommonest cause of hyperadrenocorticism is a unilateral functioning drenal tumour.

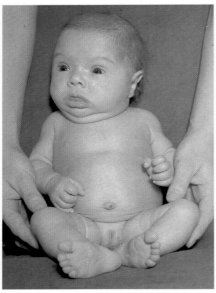

Fig. 89 Congenital hypothyroidism (cretinism). This infant has macroglossia, course facies and a short, thick neck. The hands and feet are broad and a small umbilical hernia is present. The skin is thickened and cool, and this infant had a hoarse cry. Early thyroxine replacement reduces or prevents the associated mental retardation.

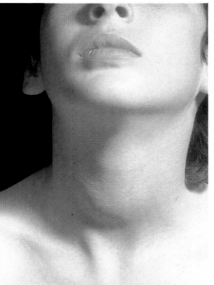

Fig. 90 Adolescent goitre. Diffuse enlargement of the thyroid gland is present in this euthyroid girl. A goitre in female adolescents usually resolves spontaneously but may be caused by autoimmune thyroiditis or dietary iodine deficiency.

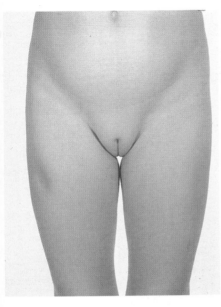

Fig. 91 Diabetic lipo-atrophy. Atrophy of subcutaneous fat at the site of repeated insulin injections is present. Continued use of such sites leads to poor diabetic control.

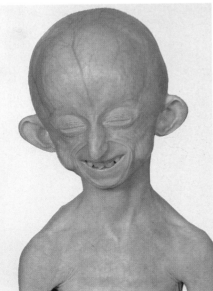

Fig. 92 Progeria. This rare disorder is characterised by premature senility. Alopecia, loss of subcutaneous fat and skeletal hypoplasia and degeneration are present. Intelligence is usually normal and death in the second decade of life from widespread atherosclerosis is common.

Metabolic Disorders

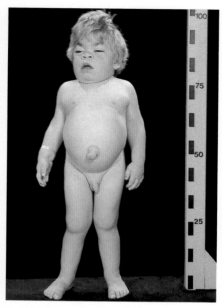

Fig. 93 Hurler's syndrome (gargoylism). This is an autosomal recessively inherited mucopolysaccharidosis (Type I). The head is large, with a flat nasal bridge and wide nostrils. The tongue is enlarged and the neck is short. The thorax is deformed, with rib splaying and hepatosplenomegaly results in abdominal distension. An umbilical hernia, genu valgum and claw hands are present and the child is mentally retarded.

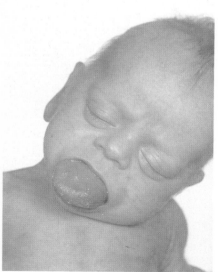

Fig. 94 Macroglossia. The tongue of this infant is grossly enlarged and cannot be accommodated in the oral cavity. Macroglossia may be a feature of hypothyroidism, mucopolysaccharidoses or Beckwith's sydrome.

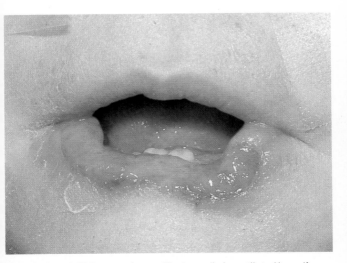

Fig. 95 Lesch-Nyhan syndrome. The lower lip is mutilated by self-destructive biting. This is an X-linked disorder of purine metabolism characterised by hyperuricaemia, mental retardation, self-mutilation, choreoathetosis and pyramidal signs.

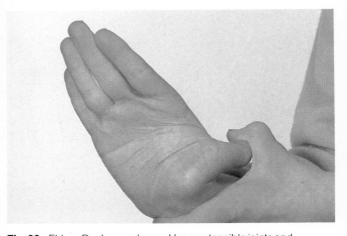

Fig. 96 Ehlers-Danlos syndrome. Hyperextensible joints and hyperelastic skin are present. This is an autosomal dominant disorder resulting in the formation of abnormal collagen. The blood vessels and skin are very fragile; the skin is easily injured and heals with 'tissue-paper' scars.

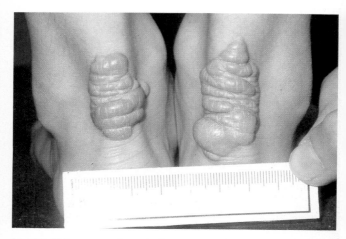

Fig. 97 Tuberose xanthomata. Lumpy cutaneous lesions are present over the Achilles tendons. They may also be found on the elbows, knees, knuckles and toes and may cause discomfort and impaired function. These lesions occur in hyperlipoproteinaemias, particularly hypercholesterolaemia.

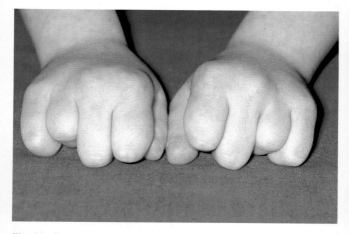

Fig. 98 Pseudohypoparathyroidism. The fingers, thumbs and hands are short and stubby. The fourth metacarpal is particularly short and the knuckle is replaced by a dimple. Characteristically hypocalcaemia, hyperphosphataemia, mental abnormalities, short stature and obesity are present. Inheritance follows an autosomal dominant or sex-linked pattern.

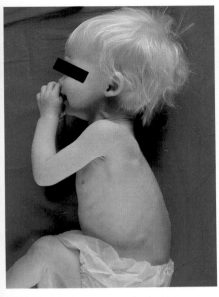

Fig. 99 Cystinosis. This fair-haired child is miserable, failing to thrive and has enlarged costochondral junctions ('rickety rosary') and wrists due to vitamin D resistant rickets. Intracellular cystine accumulation results in renal tubular damage and the Fanconi syndrome.

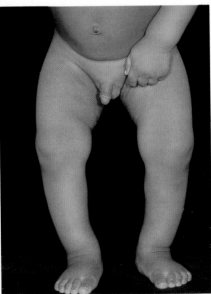

Fig. 100 Rickets. Bow legs (genu varum) and swelling of the wrist due to widening of the epiphyses are present. Nutritional rickets occurs most frequently in toddlers. Other features include a 'rickety rosary' (see Fig. 99), chest deformities, a persistent anterior fontanelle and a thin, soft cranium.

The Skin

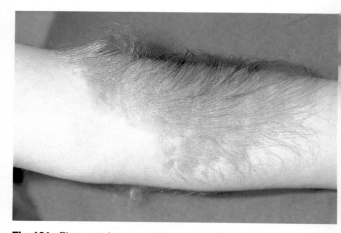

Fig. 101 Pigmented naevus. A brown macule containing hair follicles and hair is present. Pigmented naevi vary in size, shape and degree of pigmentation, may be flat or raised, with or without hair, and may occur on any part of the body. Malignant change is rare and is confined to deeply pigmented lesions.

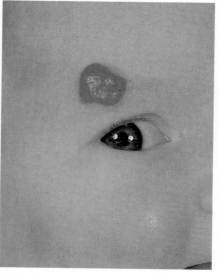

Fig. 102 Superficial cavernous haemangioma (strawberry naevus). This is a soft red lump which develops during the first month of life and may enlarge rapidly during the first year. They are common, particularly on the head, but usually resolve spontaneously.

51

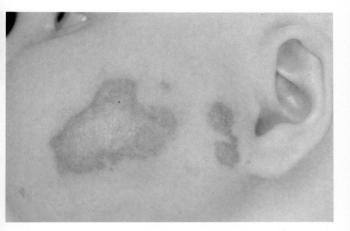

Fig. 103 Resolving superficial cavernous haemangioma. After one year of age the strawberry naevus usually starts to fade, becoming flatter and dull-red in colour.

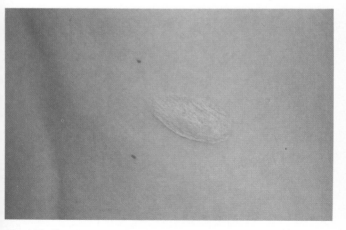

Fig. 104 Resolved superficial cavernous haemangioma. By the age of five years these lesions have usually disappeared, although a faint colouring or puckering of the skin may remain. Early surgery or freezing of growing lesions is likely to result in increased scarring.

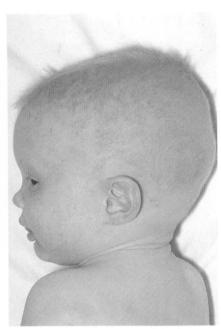

Fig. 105 Ectodermal dysplasia. The skin is dry and the hair is sparse with absent eyebrows and sparse eyelashes. There may be partial or complete absence of sweat glands leading to heat intolerance. The teeth may be hypoplastic (see Fig. 160).

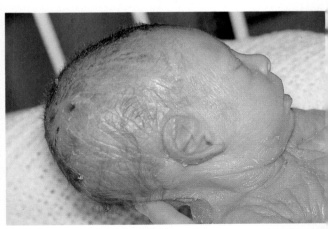

Fig. 106 Ichthyosis (ichthyosiform erythroderma). The skin is thickened, dry and a collodian-like covering is peeling off in scales. Several forms of ichthyosis exist, with varying prognoses.

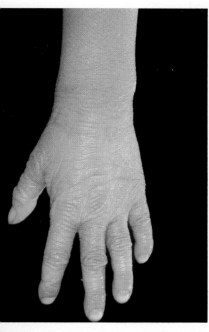

Fig. 107 Ichthyosis vulgaris. The skin is thickened, dry and fissured due to hyperkeratosis. Management is directed at maintenance of skin hydration with emulsifying ointments.

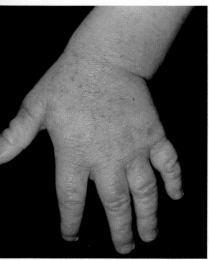

Fig. 108 Eczema. The skin is dry and thickened with erythematous papules and vesicles. The eruption is itchy and scratching may lead to secondary infection. Other atopic features are common.

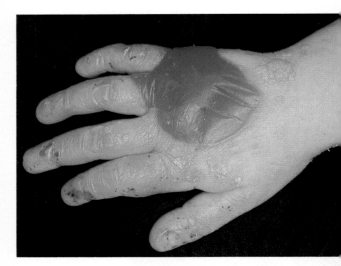

Fig. 109 Epidermolysis bullosa. A large haemorrhagic bulla is present. The skin is thin, atrophic and scarred and there is partial loss of the finger nails. This patient has the rare, recessively inherited polydysplastic type, which has a poor prognosis. Dominantly inherited forms have a much milder course.

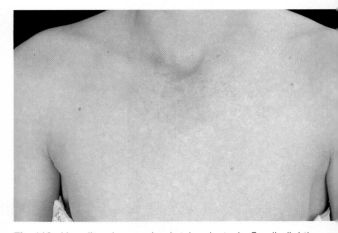

Fig. 110 Hereditary haemorrhagic telangiectasia. Small, slightly elevated red lesions are present which blanch on pressure. Similar lesions may occur on the face, lips, hands, on the mucosal surfaces of the gastrointestinal and urinary tracts, and in the brain.

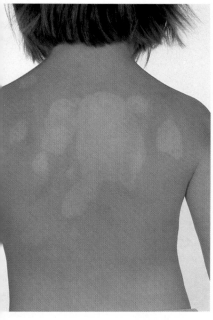

Fig. 111 Vitiligo. Well-demarcated patches of depigmentation are seen, some of which have fused together. Autoimmune disorders occur with increased frequency.

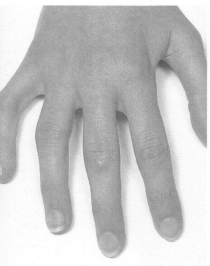

Fig. 112 Juvenile rheumatoid arthritis. A firm, non-tender subcutaneous nodule is present over the extensor tendons of the third digit. The interphalangeal joints are swollen and limitation of movement has led to muscle wasting, particularly of the first dorsal interosseus muscle.

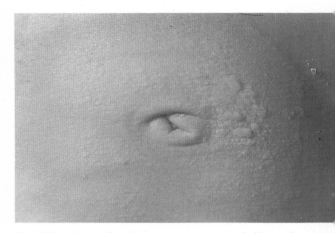

Fig. 113 Urticaria. Pale, itchy weals are surrounded by erythema. This usually occurs as an acute allergic response but may be chronic and idiopathic.

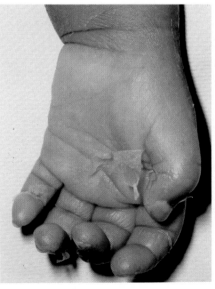

Fig. 114 Kawasaki disease. This child has exfoliation of sheets of skin from the fingers and palms. This is a late feature of the mucocutaneous lymph node syndrome which is characterised by prolonged high fever conjunctivitis, stomatitis, lymphadenopathy and erythematous rashes including the palms and soles. Myocarditis and coronary arterial aneurysms occur. Mortality is 1-2%.

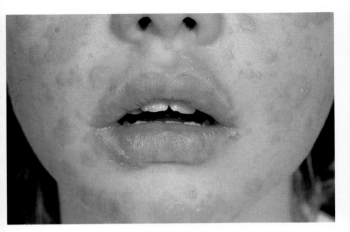

Fig. 115 Erythema multiforme. Red papules and plaques are present, many of which have become vesicular. Lesions, including a bulla, are seen around the lips, but the mucous membranes are spared. The aetiology is usually unknown but may be related to drugs, or infections including herpes simplex and mycoplasma.

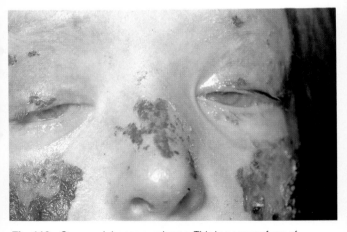

Fig. 116 Stevens Johnson syndrome. This is a severe form of erythema multiforme with involvement of the eyes, mouth and genitalia. There is ulceration and crusting of the skin at sites of bullous lesions. The eyelids are oedematous with a purulent conjunctivitis and corneal oedema.

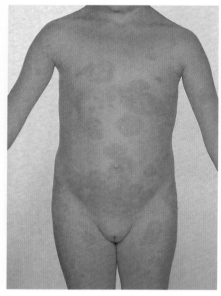

Fig. 117 Erythema marginatum. Numerous erythematous rings with pale centres of normal skin are present on the trunk and limbs. Some of these lesions have coalesced to form an irregular and changing pattern. This rash is an occasional feature of rheumatic fever.

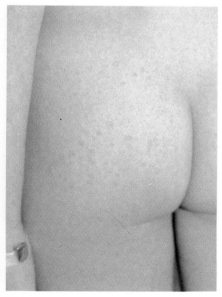

Fig. 118 Still's disease rash. There are small pale pink macules on the trunk and limbs. As in erythema marginatum, the lesions may have pale centres and change hour by hour, but are much smaller in comparison. This rash may precede the development of arthritis. By courtesy of Dr. P. Daish.

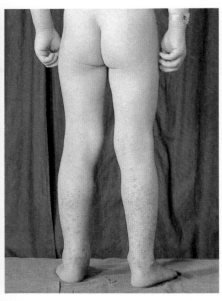

Fig. 119 Henoch-Schönlein purpura. There is a purpuric rash affecting the lower limbs. This begins as an urticarial rash which becomes purpuric and affects mainly the limbs and buttocks. There may be involvement of the gastrointestinal and renal tracts and the joints.

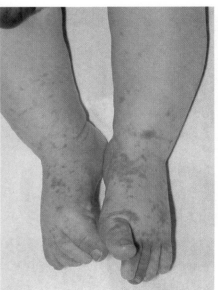

Fig. 120 Henoch-Schönlein purpura. The purpuric rash is again shown, but appears more blotchy and urticarial on the extensor surfaces near the ankle joints. The dorsal surfaces of both feet are swollen. Similar swelling may be seen on the hands and face.

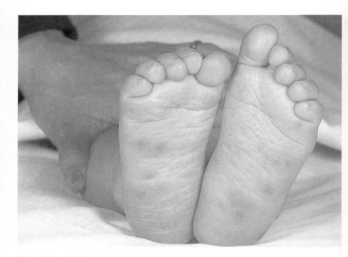

Fig. 121 Chilblains (perniosis). These are bluish-red, slightly oedematous lesions on the soles of the feet. On warming they become itchy and burning. Chilblains occur after cold exposure and are more common when the peripheries are cold as a result of conditions such as acrocyanosis.

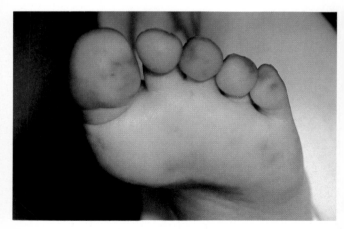

Fig. 122 Subacute bacterial endocarditis. Tender erythematous nodules are present in the pads of the toes and sole of the foot. Antibiotic prophylaxis for dental and other procedures is required in congenital heart disease, particularly ventricular septal defect and persistent ductus arteriosus, in order to prevent this condition.

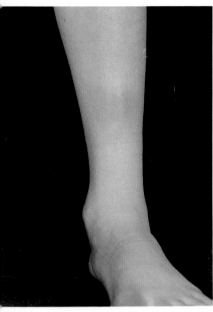

Fig. 123 Erythema nodosum. A bright red, tender, diffuse swelling is present on the shin. This will fade over several days to leave brownish staining. The lesion is seen in streptococcal infections, tuberculosis, sarcoidosis, Crohn's disease, ulcerative colitis and following sulphonamides.

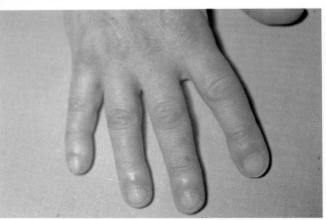

Fig. 124 Dermatomyositis. Patches of erythema with subcutaneous induration are present over the joints of the hand. This developed gradually with accompanying weakness and tenderness of the proximal muscles, and facial erythema. Dermatomyosis usually has a poor prognosis in childhood.

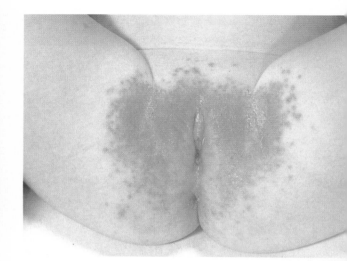

Fig. 125 Cutaneous candidiasis (thrush). A well demarcated, moist, erythematous rash, surrounded by scattered satellite lesions is present on the perineum. These features, together with the lack of sparing of skin folds and the possible presence of oral candidiasis help to distinguish this from ammoniacal dermatitis clinically.

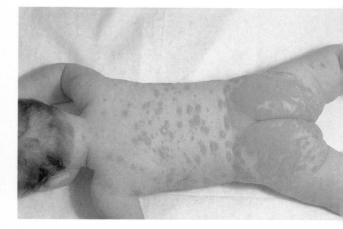

Fig. 126 Napkin psoriasis. A dry, scaly, psoriatic eruption of the napkin area, with smaller lesions on the trunk is present in this young infant. Candidal infection may be present. Spontaneous resolution occurs and there is no predisposition to psoriasis in later life.

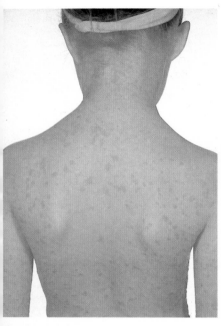

Fig. 127 Guttate psoriasis. Round, erythematous, scaly patches are present on the extensor surfaces of the arms and on the trunk and scalp. Scraping the lesions produces silvery scales. This acute form of psoriasis clears in three months but most children develop chronic psoriasis, often years later.

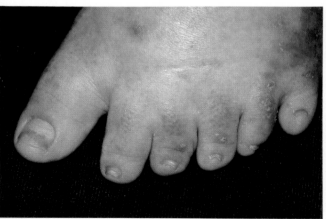

Fig. 128 Psoriasis. Nail involvement ranges from pitting (best seen on the first toe nail) to the more florid dysplastic changes shown here. Scaly skin lesions are also seen here, but nail involvement may be the only manifestation of psoriasis.

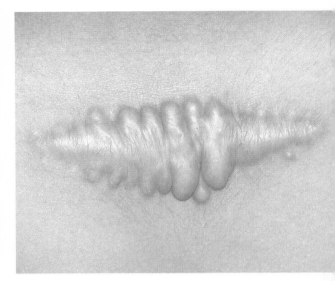

Fig. 129 Keloid. A firm, exuberant growth of fibrous scar tissue is present at the site of a surgical incision. Keloid formation in the dermis at the site of scars tends to be familial and the lesions may be pruritic or tender, often enlarging with time.

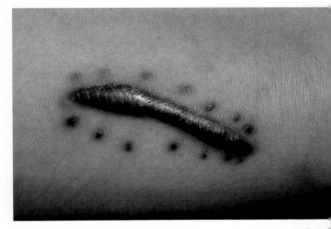

Fig. 130 Keloid. Keloid formation is more common in negroes. Small lesions may respond to the local injection of triamcinolone or cryotherapy.

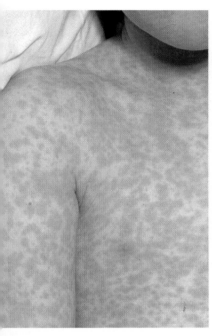

Fig. 131 Drug-induced rash. Florid erythematous macules are present. They are confluent in places and resemble the rash of measles. Urticaria, photosensitivity, erythema multiforme and exfoliative dermatitis are amongst the other dermatological manifestations of drug sensitivity. Sulphonamides and antibiotics are most commonly incriminated.

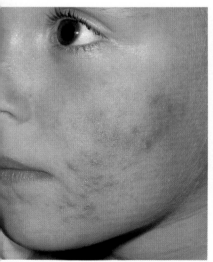

Fig. 132 Acneiform eruption following steroids. The skin of the cheek is inflamed, with pustular lesions resulting from long-term treatment with systemic steroids. Topical application of steroids may result in atrophic changes in the skin with striae, thinning and dilatation of superficial blood vessels.

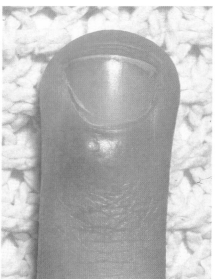

Fig. 133 Herpetic whitlow. A painful, red, paronychial swelling is present. Herpes simplex virus may be introduced from oral infections (see Fig. 134) or minor trauma. Regional lymphadenitis and malaise may be present. The lesions usually resolve spontaneously within two to three weeks.

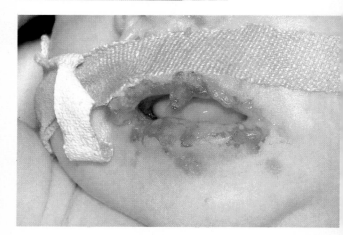

Fig. 134 Herpetic stomatitis. A florid, painful, ulcerating vesicular eruption is present on the lips and usually in the mouth causing difficulty with fluid intake. Fever, malaise and regional lymphadenopathy occur. The lesions disappear within two weeks.

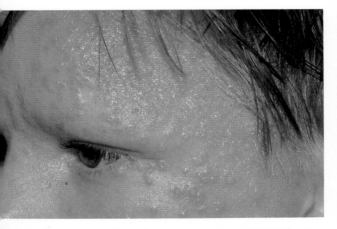

Fig. 135 Eczema herpeticum. A vesicular eruption is present due to herpes simplex infection of eczematous skin. Crops of vesicles, which may become confluent, appear over several days, accompanied by fever and malaise. Spontaneous resolution occurs over three to four weeks, but severe cases may be fatal.

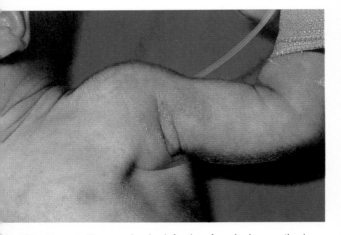

Fig. 136 Neonatal herpes simplex infection. A vesicular eruption is present on an erythematous base. The infection is acquired from vaginal delivery or prolonged rupture of membranes in a mother with genital herpes. It presents after a few days with a septicaemic-like illness which may be fatal.

68

Infectious Diseases

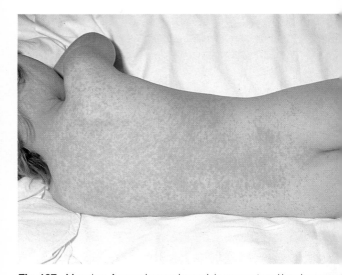

Fig. 137 Measles. A maculopapular rash is present and has become confluent along the hairline, which is where the eruption begins. The rash begins to resolve after three days leaving a brownish staining of the skin which persists for a few days.

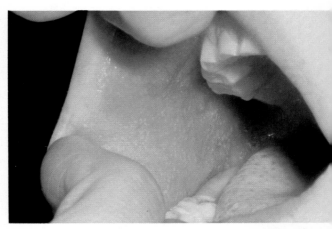

Fig. 138 Measles: Koplik's spots. Numerous small white lesions are present on the buccal mucosa. Koplik's spots are pathognomonic and are best seen during the prodromal phase of measles when fever, rhinorrhoea, conjunctivitis and coughing occur.

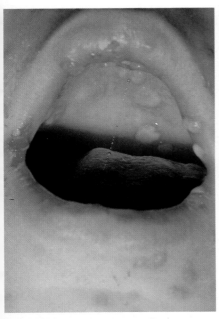

Fig. 139
Chickenpox (varicella). Following a short prodrome, crops of red papules appear, which rapidly become round, superficial, pruritic vesicles with an erythematous margin. Over three days the vesicles become pustular then form crusts and new crops may develop. Oral lesions are commonly seen.

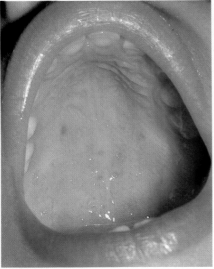

Fig. 140 Infectious mononucleosis (glandular fever). Palatal petechiae are present. They are commonly seen in infectious mononucleosis but are not pathognomonic. Fever, exudative tonsillitis, generalised lymphadenopathy, splenomegaly and a skin eruption may also be present.

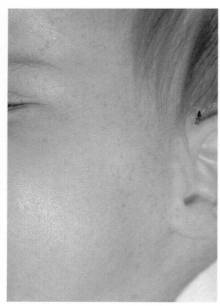

Fig. 141 Petechiae
Flat, small, superficial
haemorrhages in the
skin which do not
blanch on pressure,
are present on the
forehead and cheek.
Lesions confined to
the head and neck
can result from
screaming, vomiting
or choking, but may
be associated with
thrombocytopenia or
meningococcal
infection.

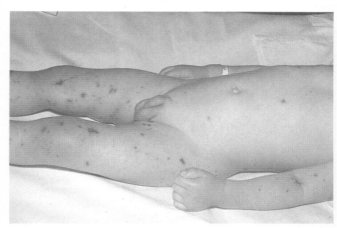

Fig. 142 Meningococcal septicaemia. A purpuric rash particularly
affecting the limbs is present in this child with an acute febrile illness
suggesting meningococcaemia. This may be followed by meningitis
or associated with a more fulminating course, characterised by
circulatory collapse and adrenal haemorrhage.

71

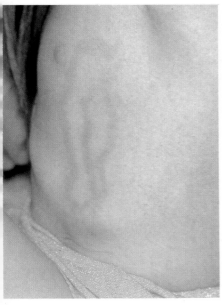

Fig. 143
Lymphangitis.
Inflammation of the
lymphatics draining
from a septic skin
lesion is present. The
lymphatics and the
regional axillary
lymph nodes are often
tender. Cat scratch
fever may also
produce such
appearances.

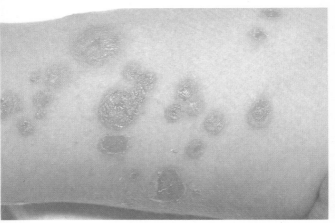

Fig. 144 Bullous impetigo. Circular, superficial bullous lesions are
present, some of which have ruptured and formed crusts or superficial
ulcers. Some lesions show central clearing. The lesions are due to a
superficial infection of the skin by *Staphylococcus aureus* or
ß-haemolytic streptococci.

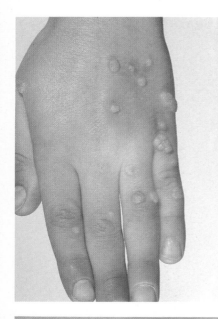

Fig. 145 Warts. Flattened, hyperkeratotic lesions are present on the hands. They are very common in children and adolescents and the majority resolve spontaneously. The most effective treatment is freezing with liquid nitrogen.

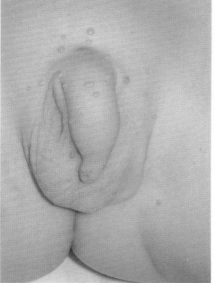

Fig. 146 Molluscum contagiosum. Small papules with central umbilication are present and are a result of a viral infection. The lesions may be found anywhere on the skin except the palms and soles, and are frequently grouped on opposing skin folds.

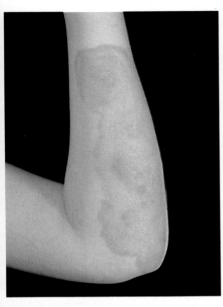

Fig. 147 Tinea corporis (ringworm). A slowly spreading, scaly, erythematous lesion is present on the arm, due to a fungal infection. The spreading edge of the lesion is inflamed and the centre of the lesion is clearing giving a characteristic ringed appearance.

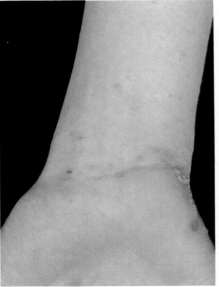

Fig. 148 Scabies. An intensely pruritic papular eruption is present on the wrist and palm due to an infestation with *Sarcoptes scabiei*. A diagnostic burrow is seen on the surface of the skin of the palm. In addition, the interdigital skin was involved. The genitalia, abdomen, axillae and, in infants, the face may be affected. Secondary infection and excoriation may obscure the diagnosis.

The Nails

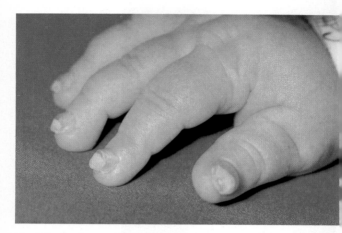

Fig. 149 Pachyonychia. The nails are overgrown, discoloured and hard. This is a rare congenital hyperkeratosis which may also involve the palms, soles, lips and tongue. Bullous skin eruptions may occur at the peripheries.

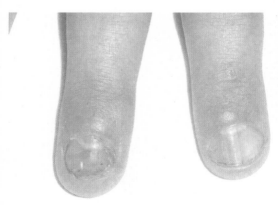

Fig. 150 Nail dystrophy. In contrast to pachyonychia, the nails are underdeveloped, thin and fragmented with longitudinal ridging. This may be an isolated finding but may be associated with other abnormalities of ectoderm or mucous membranes.

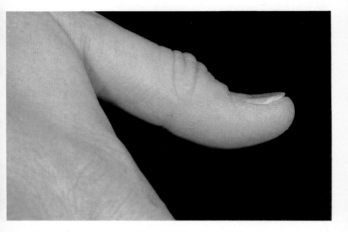

Fig. 151 Koilonychia. The nail is concave longitudinally and transversely such that a drop of water would remain upon it. This abnormality is seen in severe iron deficiency, but less commonly in children than in adults.

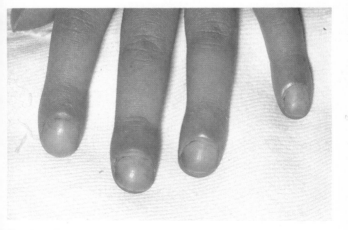

Fig. 152 Clubbing. The nails are broad and curved both longitudinally and transversely and there is loss of the angle of the nail. This patient had congenital cyanotic heart disease. Clubbing may also be seen in chronic pulmonary, bowel and liver diseases.

The Hair

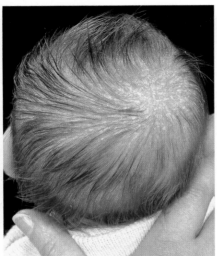

Fig. 153
Seborrhoeic dermatitis.
An area of the scalp is covered by yellow, crusted plaques (cradle cap). A similar eruption may be present on the face, trunk and in the napkin area (see Fig. 17). The lesions commonly appear in the first two months of life and clear spontaneously.

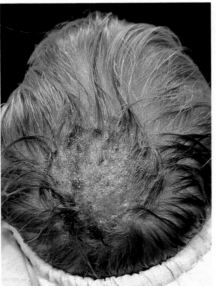

Fig. 154 Congenital aplasia of the skin. The scalp lesion is due to developmental absence of skin and hair. Small lesions may spontaneously epithelialise, but large lesions require surgery. Infection and haemorrhage may complicate this defect.

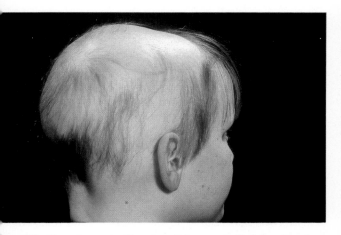

Fig. 155 Alopecia areata. There is well demarcated hair loss from the scalp, and the skin of the scalp appears normal. In extending lesions, broken hair stumps are seen. Most cases recover from a first attack.

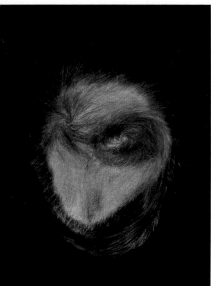

Fig. 156
Trichotillomania. The area of hair loss is irregular and may migrate with regrowing stubble at the edges. This is produced by repetitive twisting or pulling of the hair and may be a sign of emotional disturbance.

The Teeth

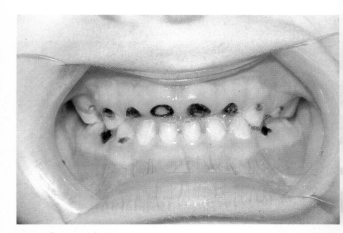

Fig. 157 Dental caries. Extensive tooth decay is present in this 6 year old child. Factors predisposing to such advanced caries include low dietary fluoride intake, high sucrose intake, poor oral hygiene, enamel hypoplasia and poor parenting.

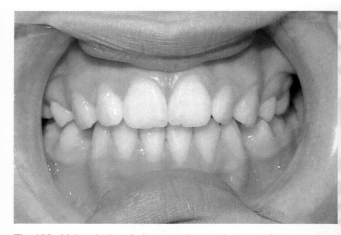

Fig. 158 Malocclusion. An increased space is present between the upper and lower anterior teeth due to the cusps of the posterior mandibular teeth being behind and inside the cusps of the corresponding maxillary teeth. Facial growth may be affected and tooth loss in later life is more common.

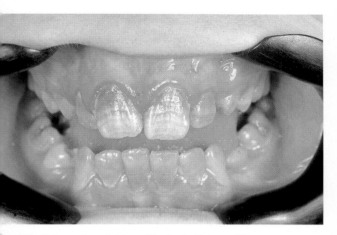

Fig. 159 Tetracycline staining of the teeth. Tetracyclines are incorporated into teeth and bones causing yellowish-brown discoloration of the teeth if administered during the periods of enamel formation. For primary dentition this is from the fourth month of intrauterine life to the tenth month of life, and for permanent dentition it is from the fourth month of life to the age of sixteen.

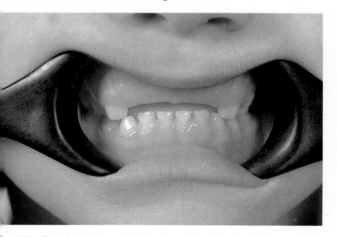

Fig. 160 Ectodermal dysplasia (see Fig. 105). Small, widely spaced or absent teeth are a feature of ectodermal dysplasia. This may also be seen in pseudohypoparathyroidism, and other disorders.

The Tongue

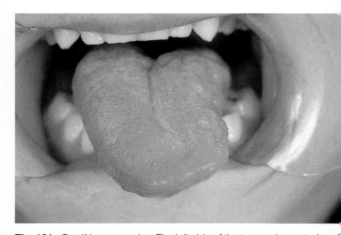

Fig. 161   Twelfth nerve palsy. The left side of the tongue is wasted and fasiculating as a result of a lower motor neurone lesion. On protrusion, the tongue is pushed to the left. Unilateral lesions may be due to congenital abnormalities of the foramen magnum, poliomyelitis, tuberculous meningitis or tumour.

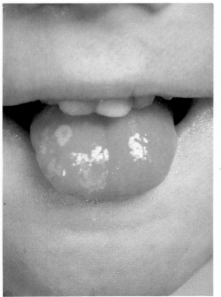

Fig. 162   Oral candidiasis (thrush) (see also Fig. 125). Adherent white patches are present on the tongue, due to an infection with *Candida albicans*. Infection is common in the newborn, and during antibiotic or corticosteroid therapy. Chronic infection may occur in impaired immunity states and in hypoparathyroidism.

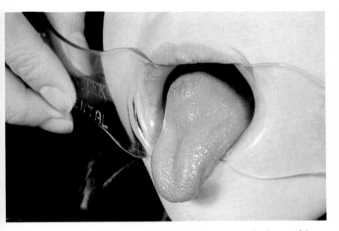

Fig. 163 Lingual thyroid gland. A mass is present at the base of the tongue, comprising thyroid tissue which has failed to descend to its normal anatomical position. In some cases, the entire thyroid gland may fail to descend.

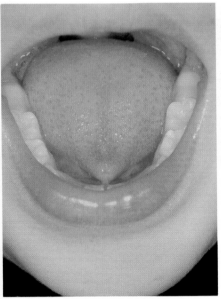

Fig. 164 Tongue tie (ankyloglossia). A short lingual frenum is present which extends to the tip of the tongue, and prevents tongue protrusion. Surgical intervention is seldom necessary as this anomaly is rarely responsible for difficulties in sucking or speech.

Non-accidental Injury

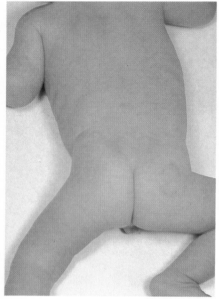

Fig. 165 Bite marks. Bite marks are present on the buttock of this infant corresponding in size and shape to those produced by an adult's teeth. These must be distinguished from bites by siblings.

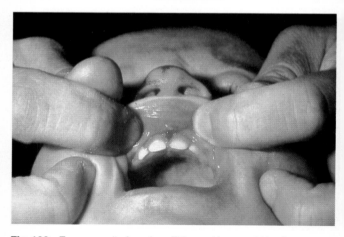

Fig. 166 Torn upper lip frenulum. This must be sought in all suspected cases of non-accidental injury, although it may be acquired accidentally.

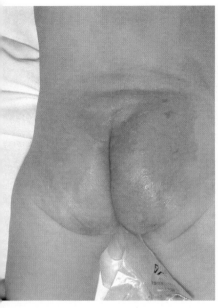

Fig. 167 Scald. The skin of this infant is scalded as a result of forced contact with hot water. Scalding confined to the buttocks and back suggests that the infant may have been lowered into bath water known to be too hot.

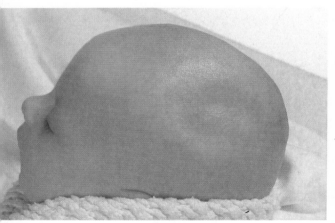

Fig. 168 Skull fracture. An obviously depressed skull fracture is present in this two month old infant. In a child of this age this is highly suspicious of non-accidental injury. Radiological examination of the skeleton for other fractures is mandatory in suspected cases of non-accidental injury in infants and toddlers.

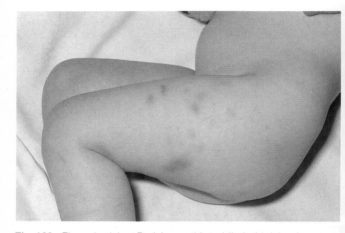

Fig. 169 Finger bruising. Bruising on this toddler's thigh has been caused by forceful gripping between the fingers and thumb of one hand. Widespread bruising, over and above that normally seen on the shins of toddlers, particularly if in unusual sites, strongly suggests non-accidental injury.

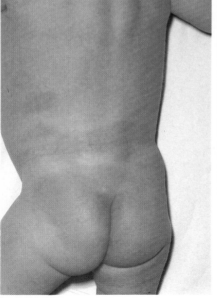

Fig. 170 Mongolian blue spot. Well demarcated areas of slate-blue pigmentation are common on the buttocks and back of non-Caucasian infants. They become less obvious as skin pigmentation slowly increases with time and should be distinguished from the widespread bruising sometimes seen in non-accidental injury.

Malignant Disease and Haematology

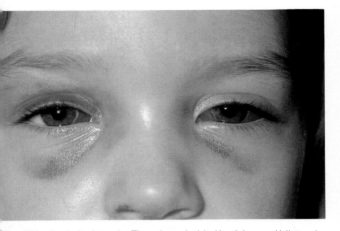

Fig. 171 Acute leukaemia. There is periorbital bruising and bilateral subconjunctival haemorrhage resulting from thrombocytopaenia due to acute leukaemia. Fundoscopy may reveal retinal haemorrhages and leukaemic exudates.

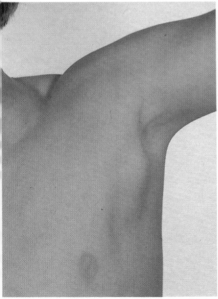

Fig. 172 Acute leukaemia. A large, discrete, painless, rubbery lymph gland is present in the axilla. There was no evidence of sepsis in the area drained by the gland. Lymphadenopathy elsewhere and hepatosplenomegaly were present in this child with acute leukaemia.

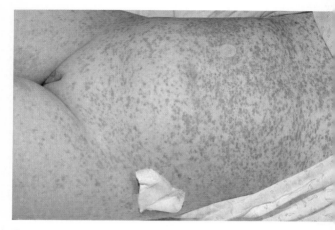

Fig. 173 Idiopathic thrombocytopaenic purpura. Multiple spontaneous haemorrhages into the skin have resulted in macular lesions which do not blanche on pressure. There is a dressing over the site of an iliac crest bone marrow aspiration, which was performed to exclude leukaemia and aplastic anaemia as causes of the thrombocytopaenia before beginning steroid therapy.

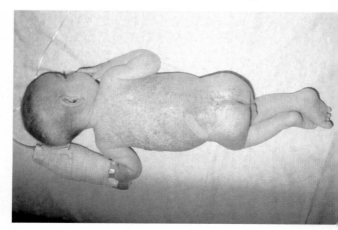

Fig. 174 Histiocytosis X. This infant is pale with a widespread rash consisting of purpuric and infiltrated seborrhoeic dermatitis-like lesions. This rash is characteristic of Letterer Siwe disease, which is a variant of histiocytosis X occurring in early childhood and infancy.

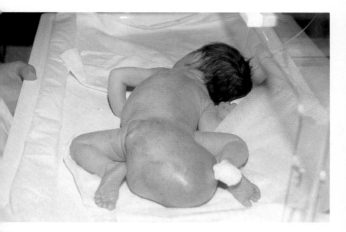

Fig. 175 Sacrococcygeal teratoma. There is a large mass arising from the coccyx of this newborn baby girl. This is the commonest form of teratoma and is usually present at birth. Many are non-malignant and can be completely excised.

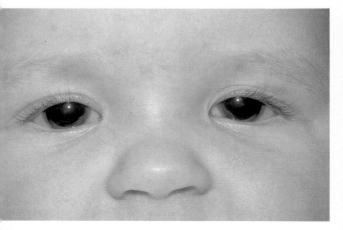

Fig. 176 Aniridia. The irises are hypoplastic. Nephroblastoma (Wilm's tumour) may be associated with sporadic aniridia and other developmental malformations including hemihypertrophy. Familial aniridia is associated with other ocular abnormalities.

The Gastrointestinal Tract

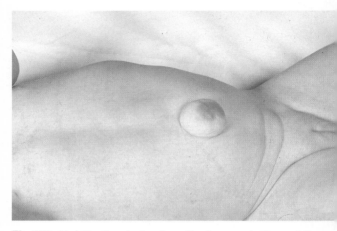

Fig. 177 Umbilical hernia. A soft swelling is present at the umbilicus. It enlarges with crying but is fully reducible. Umbilical herniae are particularly common in negro infants. Most close spontaneously by the age of five. Rarely, surgery is necessary for persistent herniae or strangulation.

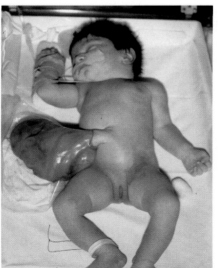

Fig. 178
Exomphalos. The abdominal contents are herniated at the umbilicus into a sac comprising peritoneum and amnion. One-third of these infants are born pre-term and other congenital abnormalities may be present, including Beckwith's syndrome (see Fig. 12).

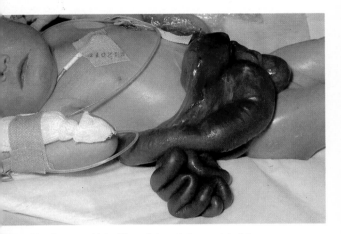

Fig. 179 Gastroschisis. There is herniation and, in this case, strangulation of the bowel through a small, full thickness defect in the anterior abdominal wall. No sac is present so fluid losses must be minimised by covering the bowel with polythene.

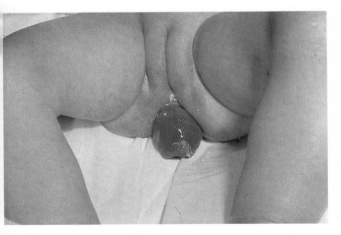

Fig. 180 Rectal prolapse. This may be associated with cystic fibrosis, malnutrition or paralysis of the muscles of the pelvic floor (e.g. in spina bifida). Repeated recurrence following manual reduction may require submucosal injection of sclerosant. By courtesy of Prof. L. Spitz.

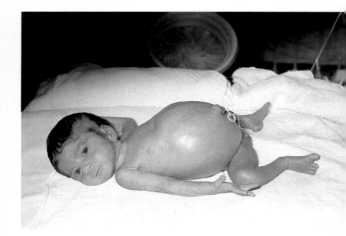

Fig. 181 Functional intestinal obstruction. Gross abdominal distension is present without a physical obstruction. This child had watery diarrhoea from birth, with stool chloride exceeding the sum of sodium and potassium concentrations due to a defect in intestinal chloride transport – congenital chloridorrhoea. Pseudo-obstruction may also be produced by muscular and neuronal disorders of the gut.

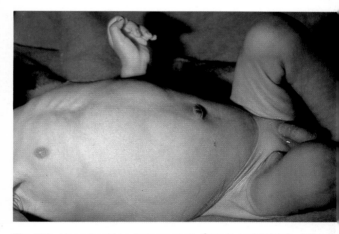

Fig. 182 Hypertrophic pyloric stenosis. Gastric peristalsis is visible in the left upper quadrant in a dehydrated infant. Non bile-stained, projectile vomiting begins in the first few weeks of life and a palpable pyloric tumour may be present during a feed. By courtesy of Prof. L Spitz.

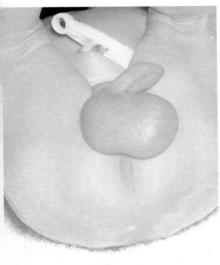

Fig. 183 Rectal atresia. The normal anal opening is absent and replaced by a small depression. The rectum ends blindly in the pelvis, above the levator ani muscle. Associated anomalies are often present, particularly of the upper urinary tract. A left hydrocoele is also present.

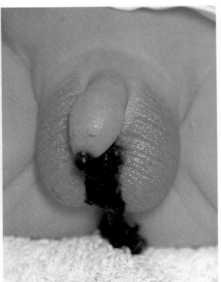

Fig. 184 Rectovesical fistula. Meconium has been passed per urethra in this newborn infant with rectal atresia, indicating the presence of a rectourinary fistula. Fistulae into the vagina or perineum also occur.

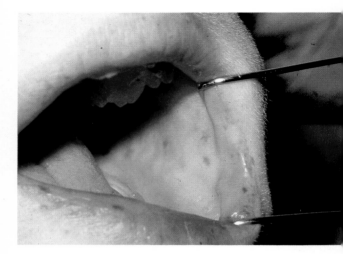

Fig. 185 Peutz Jegher's syndrome. Small patches of pigmentation develop on the lips and buccal mucosa in early childhood. Intestinal polyposis leads to abdominal pain, intussusception or bleeding but malignant change is rare. There is autosomal dominant inheritance with incomplete penetrance.

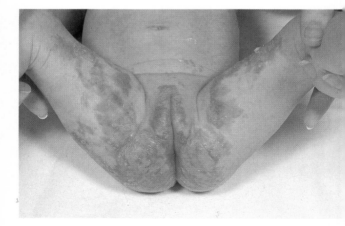

Fig. 186 Acrodermatitis enteropathica. An inherited defect of zinc absorption results in this scaly erythematous rash at mucocutaneous junctions, diarrhoea and failure to thrive. This potentially fatal disease responds dramatically to oral zinc supplements. A similar rash is seen in zinc deficiency states.

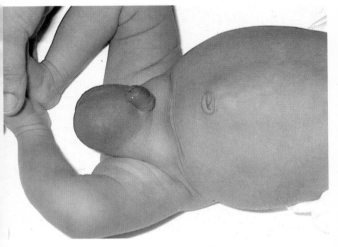

Fig. 187   Bilateral inguinal herniae. Bilateral inguinal and scrotal swellings are present as a result of herniation of abdominal contents along a patent processus vaginalis. Early herniotomy is indicated in all cases. An inguinal hernia in a female infant suggests possible testicular feminisation syndrome.

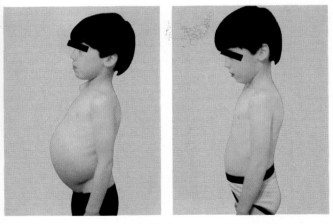

Fig. 188   Air swallowing. This child has a markedly distended abdomen during the day, but the distension is not present on waking. This is due to air swallowing and not intestinal disease and is particularly common in toddlers.

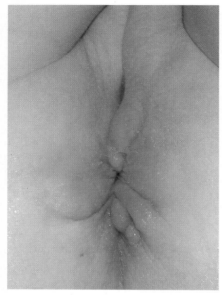

Fig. 189 Crohn's disease. The perianal area is indurated and anal fissures and skin tags are present. Crohn's disease usually presents in late childhood, often with the insidious onset of abdominal pain, diarrhoea, anaemia or growth failure.

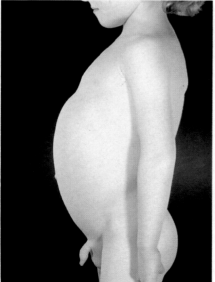

Fig. 190 Hirschprung's disease. The abdomen is markedly distended and a faecal mass was palpable in the left lower quadrant. There was a history of chronic constipation with small pellet-like or fluid stools and failure to thrive. Hirschprung's disease in the older child may be confused with malabsorption syndromes. Presentation with intestinal obstruction is common in the neonatal period.

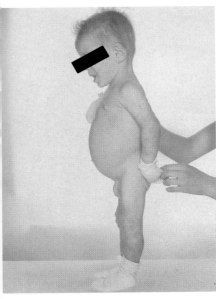

Fig. 191 Food allergy. This toddler is failing to thrive, has abdominal distention, scanty hair, eczema and diarrhoea due to cow's milk protein intolerance. A patchy enteropathy of the small intestine is usually present and symptoms respond to dietary antigen withdrawal.

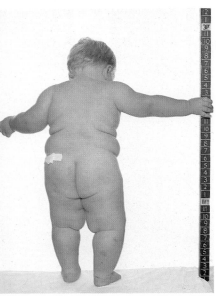

Fig. 192 Obesity. Obesity in childhood is only rarely a complication of endocrine disorders (e.g. Frohlich's syndrome, Prader-Willi syndrome). Children with simple obesity are usually of above average height. Psycho-social problems are often present in the families of grossly obese children.

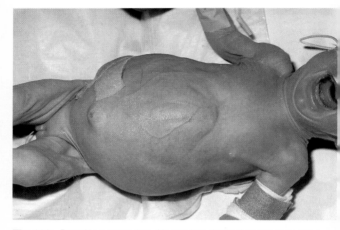

Fig. 193 Portal hypertension. Abdominal distention due to ascites, and hepatomegaly with dilated veins on the abdominal wall are present in this wasted child with chronic liver disease and portal hypertension. The dilated veins are part of a collateral circulation between the portal and systemic venous systems.

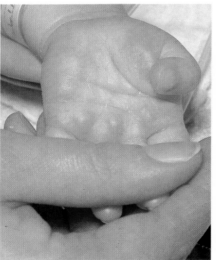

Fig. 194 Palmar erythema. This infant with chronic liver disease shows erythema of the palms, most marked over the thenar and hypothenar eminences.

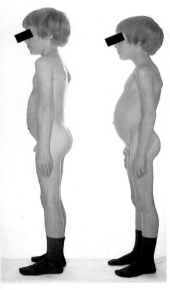

Fig. 195 Coeliac disease. The boy on the right with coeliac disease, has abdominal distention and is much shorter than his unaffected twin. Dietary gluten induces villous atrophy of the small intestine with subsequent malabsorption and growth delay, all of which respond to a gluten-free diet.

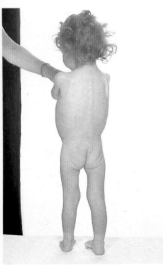

Fig. 196 Coeliac disease. This girl with coeliac disease has abdominal distention and is malnourished with marked buttock wasting. Children with coeliac disease are commonly anorexic and irritable and usually have diarrhoea or steatorrhoea.

The Locomotor System

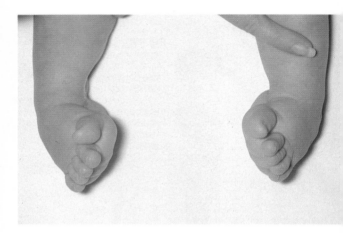

Fig. 197 Talipes equinovarus. There is plantar flexion with inversion of the ankles and inversion and adduction of the feet. Passive correction is not possible and this is a true deformity. Management of club-feet is by stretching exercises, splintage and sometimes surgery.

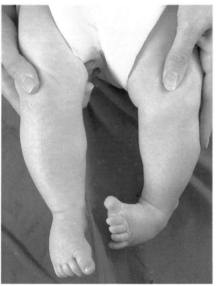

Fig. 198 Metatarsus varus. The left forefoot is medially deviated but unlike talipes, the heel is in line with the leg, and the foot can be passively flexed. Most cases resolve spontaneously by the age of four years and the remainder can be corrected at this age.

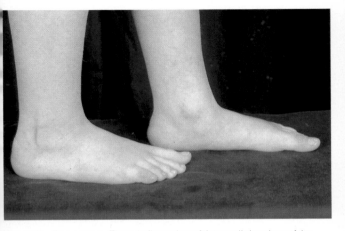

Fig. 199 Pes planus. There is flattening of the medial arches of the feet resulting in flat feet. These are usually painless and the feet are normally mobile. Insoles or supports in the shoes may be helpful. Flat feet caused by local disease, neurological disease or joint laxity require specific management.

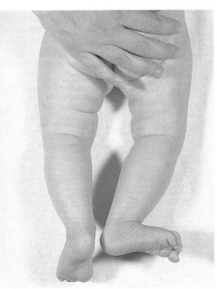

Fig. 200 External rotation of leg. There is external rotation of the right hip and lower leg of this infant, due to femoral retroversion. This abnormality which is often bilateral is usually postural and resolves when walking commences although a few cases persist. Congenital dislocation of the hip must be excluded.

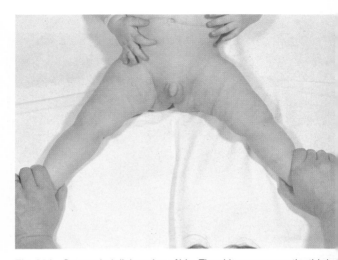

Fig. 201 Congenital dislocation of hip. The skin creases on the thighs are asymmetrical and abduction of the right hip is limited in this six month old with right CDH which was not detected in the neonatal period.

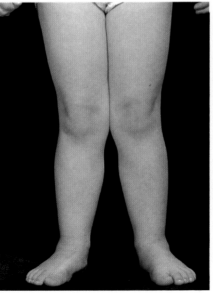

Fig. 202 Genu valgum. Knock knees are present with wide separation of the medial malleoli and, as is often associated a degree of pes planus. Underlying rickets should be considered. Nearly all cases resolve spontaneously. If intermaleolar separation is more than 9 cm when the child is lying down, orthopaedic referral is indicated.

101

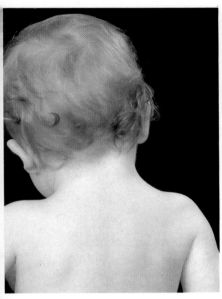

Fig. 203 Torticollis. In the neonatal period, a left sternomastoid swelling was noted. The child has subsequently had a persistent tilt of the head to the left – torticollis. Failure of improvement with physiotherapy and development of facial deformity are indications for surgical correction.

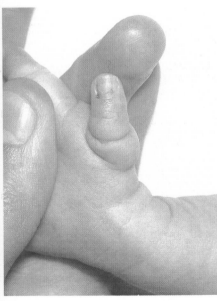

Fig. 204 Congenital ring compression. A compression ring is present around the proximal phalanx of the thumb. More severe variants may be associated with distal lymphoedema or amputation. The relationship to amniotic bands is unclear.

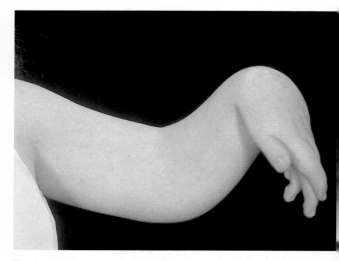

Fig. 205 Arthrogryposis. The left arm is small with fixed deformity resulting in pronation of the forearm and flexion of the wrist. This is a sporadic congenital disorder of unknown aetiology. The abnormal joints are related to weak hypoplastic muscles either neuropathic, myopathic or mixed in origin.

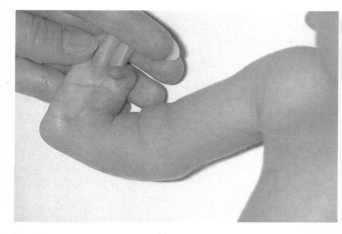

Fig. 206 Absent radius. The right radius and thumb are absent. This abnormality may be associated with cardiac defects or Fanconi pancytopaenia or with vertebral, anal, tracheoesophageal and renal defects (VATER association).

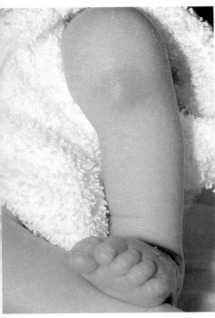

Fig. 207 Osteitis. There is swelling, erythema and tenderness below the knee of this newborn infant. The child was unwell and resented handling before these signs appeared. Staphylococci are usually found in blood culture and prompt systemic antibiotic treatment is required.

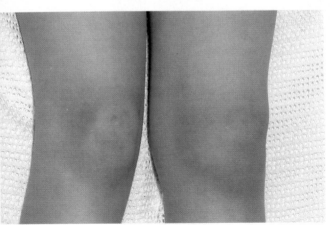

Fig. 208 Arthritis. The left knee is swollen and painful. Careful examination revealed no bony tenderness to suggest osteomyelitis. Aspiration of the joint excluded septic arthritis in this boy with Crohn's disease.

104

The Nervous System

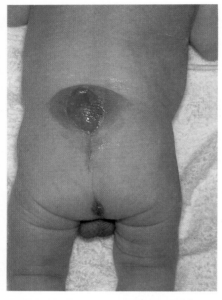

Fig. 209
Myelomeningocoele.
A bony lumbosacral
defect is present with
a sac containing CSF,
and neural tissue
protruding through
the skin. Abnormal
neurological signs are
present in the lower
limbs and sphincters,
and hydrocephalus is
commonly associated
(see Figs. 215 and
216).

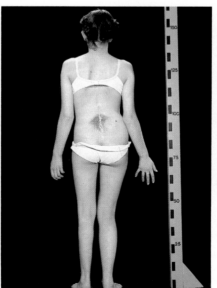

Fig. 210 Spinal
dysraphism. There is
a tuft of hair overlying
the lumbar spine, a
scoliosis and
shortening of the left
leg. A vertebral
anomaly may be
present on X-ray.
Neurological deficit
results from tethering
of the cord and
resultant traction or
from direct pressure
by a bony spur
(diastematomyelia).

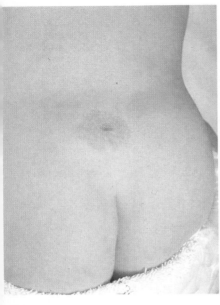

Fig. 211 Sacral sinus. A sinus is present in the midline extending from the skin to the spinal cord. Bacterial meningitis may develop and midline sinuses should always be sought at birth and in all children with bacterial meningitis. A haemangioma is also present here.

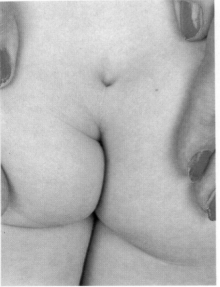

Fig. 212 Sacrococcygeal pit. A blind-ending sinus is present, overlying the sacrum. Sinuses may be present anywhere along the vertebral column. Cysts may develop in a sinus, causing neurological disturbances or abscess formation.

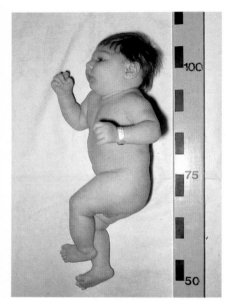

Fig. 213
Microcephaly. The vault of the skull is small, such that the ears appear disproportionately large. Cerebral hypoplasia and mental retardation commonly occur. Secondary forms may result from intrauterine infections or maternal irradiation in early pregnancy.

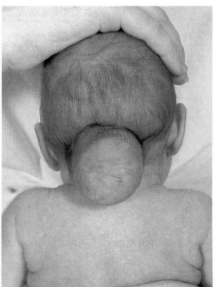

Fig. 214
Encephalocoele. A midline occipital cranial defect is present, through which the meninges and brain have herniated. The lesion may occur anteriorly. It is often complicated by neurological deficit and sometimes hydrocephalus.

107

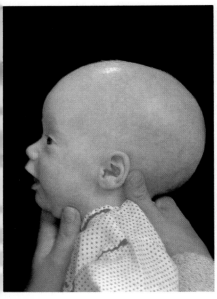

Fig. 215
Hydrocephalus. The head of this infant has progressively enlarged as a result of an excess of cerebrospinal fluid within the ventricles. The skull sutures become separated and the anterior fontanelle bulges in rapidly progressive hydrocephalus.

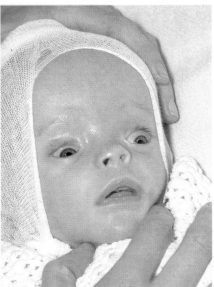

Fig. 216
Hydrocephalus. The sclera is visible above the iris in the eyes of this infant. This is due to downward deviation of the eyes in severe infantile hydrocephalus and is called the sunsetting sign. In chronic untreated cases, optic atrophy develops.

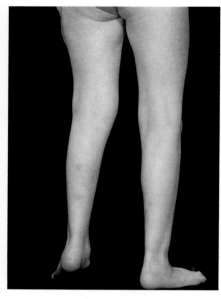

Fig. 217 Cerebral palsy. The left leg is thin and weak with a degree of circumduction and contracture at the heel. This appearance is due to cerebral palsy which results in spastic hemiplegia in approximately one-third of cases.

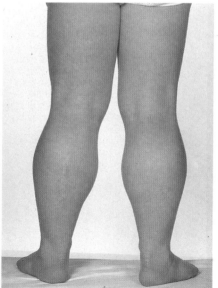

Fig. 218 Duchenne muscular dystrophy. The calf muscles are weak and hypertrophied, partly due to fatty infiltration. This is often described as pseudohypertrophic muscular dystrophy. This X-linked condition presents in boys after the age of three with difficulty climbing stairs or a waddling gait.

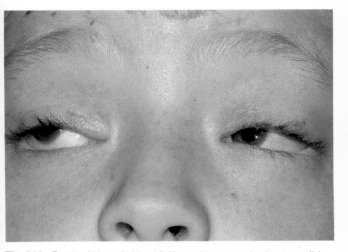

Fig. 219 Ptosis. Although this child is gazing upwards, the upper lids are not retracted. Drooping of the eyelids can be congenital or myopathic. Paralysis of the third cranial nerve or sympathetic supply (Horner's syndrome) usually causes unilateral ptosis.

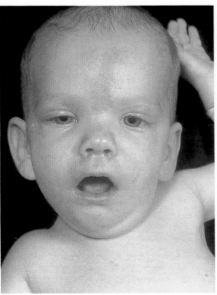

Fig. 220 Myopathic facies. There is weakness of the facial muscles resulting in bilateral ptosis, an open mouth and an expressionless face. This child has myotonic dystrophy, as did the mother who had difficulty in relaxing a hand grip.

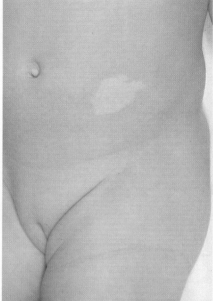

Fig. 221 Tuberose sclerosis. A well demarcated depigmented patch known as a white leaf macule is present on the trunk. Such lesions up to 3 cm in diameter, are seen from birth and may be found in asymptomatic relatives. This autosomal dominant condition may cause mental retardation and epilepsy.

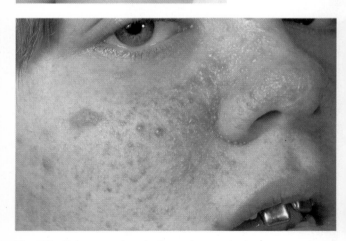

Fig. 222 Tuberose sclerosis. A papular eruption is present on the cheeks and nose of this child. The lesion is known as adenoma sebaceum but is due to angiofibromata which develop in early to mid childhood. Fibromata may also occur on the fingers, toes and gums.

111

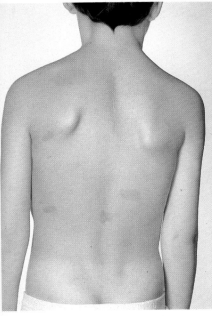

Fig. 223
Neurofibromatosis.
Several
hyperpigmented
lesions are present on
the trunk. These café
au lait patches can
occur in normal
children but six
patches greater than
1.5 cm in diameter are
considered
diagnostic of
neurofibromatosis. A
dorsal spinal
neurofibroma has
been surgically
removed.

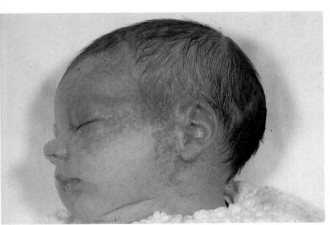

Fig. 224 Sturge Weber syndrome. A port wine stain is present in the
left trigeminal region. Associated congenital capillary haemangiomata
may involve the meninges, resulting in cortical damage which
produces convulsions, mental retardation or hemiparesis.

Index

All entries refer to Fig. numbers.